Atlas Of
NEURORADIOLOGY

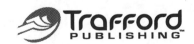
Trafford
PUBLISHING™

1663 Liberty Drive Bloomington,
IN 47403 (USA)

Order this book online at www.trafford.com
or email orders@trafford.com

Most Trafford titles are also available at major online book retailers.

Printed in the United States of America.

ISBN: 978-1-4269-6968-3 (sc)
ISBN: 978-1-4269-6971-3 (e)

Library of Congress Control Number: 2011909194

Trafford rev. 01/25/2012

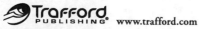 www.trafford.com

North America & International
toll-free: 1 888 232 4444 (USA & Canada)
phone: 250 383 6864 ♦ fax: 812 355 4082

Atlas of Neuroradiology
200 Cases (COMMON DISEASES)

Ammar HAOUIMI
DIS, DUCT, DURP, EDUS (France)
Consultant Radiologist
Es-Salem Imaging Center
Batna, Algeria

In Colloboration with

Rabah BOUGUELAA
DIS (France)
Consultant Radiologist
Es-Salem Imaging Center
Batna, Algeria

To

My wife and children for understanding and tolering, the countless hours
when I was behind the computer working on this book .

Preface

The invention of computed tomography and magnetic resonance imaging has completely changed the morphological and functional exploration of the nervous system and therefore has a very precise approach to diagnosis of the most neurological diseases.

The progress in neuroradiological imaging need intensive further training to enable all radiologists and clinicians, the optimal use of these techniques.

The topics covered in Atlas of Neuroradiology represent the common and important diseases encountered in neuroradiology. The material presented for each case provides a thorough and comprehensive description of the disease entity enabling the radiologist or the clinician to develop a clear concept of the entity through the different imaging modalities that are present. In this book, I attempt, al least to fill a small gap of knowledge in neuroradiology and hope that will be useful for residents in radiology, radiologists, neurologists and neurosurgeons.

Ammar HAOUIMI

Acknowledgements

I would like to acknowledge my teachers, Abdelkrim Berrah Professor and chairman, Department of Medicine at Bab El-oued University Hospital, Algiers, and Professor Moulay Ahmed Meziane, Head Section of Thoracic Imaging, Department of Diagnostic Radiology, Cleveland Clinic Fondation Ohio, USA and Professor Mosleh Al-Raddadi, Head of Radiology Department at King Fahad University Hospital Al Madinah, KSA, for their support and encouragement to continue to grow.

I am grateful for the support and friendship of my colleagues Drs Gamal Hassan, Abdullah Al-Taifi, Ridha Okbi, Abdullah Dardiri, Hussain Shahid, Mohammed Bediaf, Djamel Bourenane, Mohammed Said Gouhiri, Djamel Ouslimane, Saadeddine Yassine, Abdelkader Nashed, Abdelwahab M Gabal, Aftab Ahmed Shaikh, Nacer Kernane, Amrane Mohammedi, Mourad Chirou, Abderrahmane Bennouar, Fouad Athmani, Rabah Gourab, yasmine Bala, Soraya Benali, Souhil Abida, Farid Abed. Kamel Dahmane, Louardi Mohammedi, Toufik Nia and Mahfouth Abdmeziem.

I want to thank my family especially my parents, parents in law and my brothers Nacer, Abdelkader, Ahmed and Abdellatif for their love and support.

To Mr. Ahmed Zergui Head of CIDIS Company.

I would like to thank also all staff working in our Es-Salem Imaging Center, Samia Hocine, A Chinaz, Siham Mekaddem, Rania Lombarkia, Samia Ghenai, Nasereddine Benamor, M'hammed Bouguelaa, Ayachi Nezzar, Zoheir Mellah, Hicham Kadri, Mustapha Benguiba, Mustapha Aoura.

Finally, I would like to express my gratitude to Mr Oliver Mitchell, Supervisor Publishing Team and Mr. Dennis Taylor Publishing Services Associates at Trafford Publishing (Bloomington, USA).

Contents

Brain

-Vascular Diseases and Trauma: (Cases 1 to 34) 1

-Infection and Inflammatory Diseases: (Cases 35 to 44) 41

-White Matter and Degenerative Diseases: (Cases 45 to 46)........................55

-Intra-and extra-axial Tumors: (Cases 47 to 104) 59

-Malformations, Phacomatosis and Granulomatosis: (Cases 105 to 139) 127

Spine and Spinal Cord

-Tumors of Spine: (Cases 140 to 152) 171

-Infection and Inflammatory Diseases of Spine: (Cases 153 to 161)............187

-Degenerative, and Trauma. of spine: (Cases 162 to 174)............................199

-Congenital anomalies of Spine and Spinal Cord: (Cases 175 to 198)..........215

-Miscellaneous: (Cases 199 to 200) 243

BRAIN

VASCULAR and TRAUMATIC

Case 1

Clinical Presentation

A 49 year-old female patient with new onset of nausea, vomiting, mild left weakness, right facial numbness, vertigo, and ataxia.

Radiological Findings

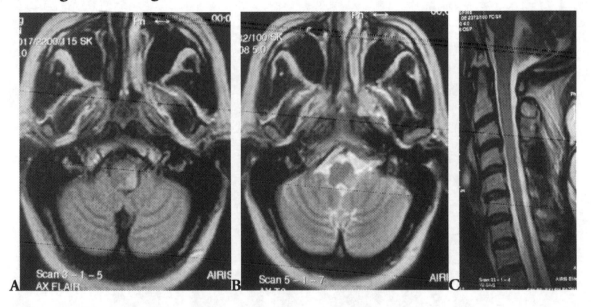

MR Scan of brain axial FLAIR (A), and T2 (B) and sagittal T2 (C) of spine show a focal high signal intensity area of the left medulla. No other abnormality of the cerebellar hemispheres or the spinal cord. This is consistent with an acute infarct in the PICA distribution.

Diagnosis: Wallenberg Syndrome

Case 2

Clinical Presentation

An 86 year-old female patient presenting an acute dizziness, vertigo, dysarthria, the 2nd nonenhanced CT Scan (C, D) was performed 48 hours later after sudden loss of consiousness, weakness of limbs and blindness.

Radiological Findings

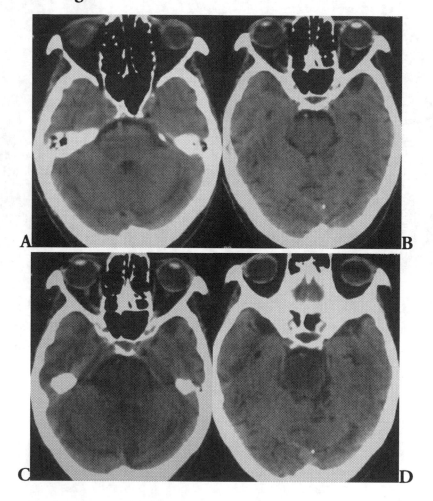

Nonenhanced brain CT Scan: The first brain CT Scan(**A, B**) done few hours after the acute onset shows normal size and density of the brainstem and both cerebellar hemispheres. The second CT Scan(**C, D**) done 48 hours later shows an enlarged brainstem with large central low-density area consisting with brainstem infarction.

Diagnosis: Brainstem Infarction

Case 3

Clinical Presentation

A 65 year-old female patient presented with left hemiplegia.

Radiological Findings

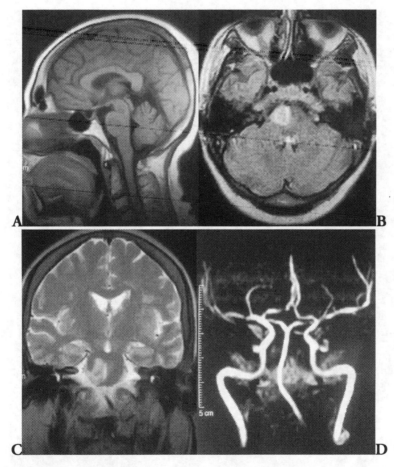

Brain MR, non-enhanced sagittal T1 (A), axial FLAIR (B), coronal T2 (C) and MRA-3D-TOF (D) showing a low-T1 and high-FLAIR and T2 lesion involving the right anterolateral aspect of the pons. The MRA shows complete thrombosis of the right vertebral artery.

Diagnosis: Brainstem Infarction

Case 4

Clinical Presentation

An 86 year-old male patient with acute diminution of the vision.

Radiological Findings

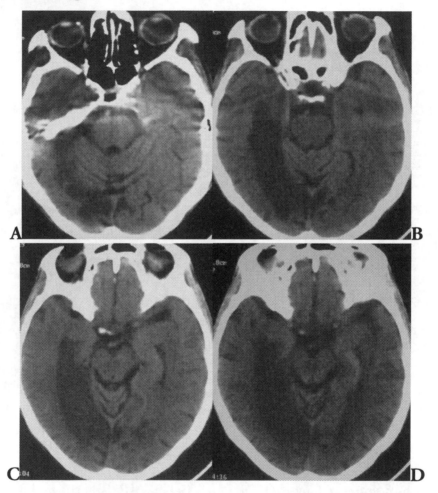

Plain brain CT Scan reveals a large low-density area in the right temporo-occipital region in the distribution of the posterior cerebral artery (PCA) territory with mass effect on the adjacent temporal horn. No other abnormality.

Diagnosis: PCA Territory Infarction

Case 5

Clinical Presentation

A 64 year-old female diabetic and hypertensive patient with one week history of temporo-spatial disorientation, headaches and drowsiness.

Radiological Findings

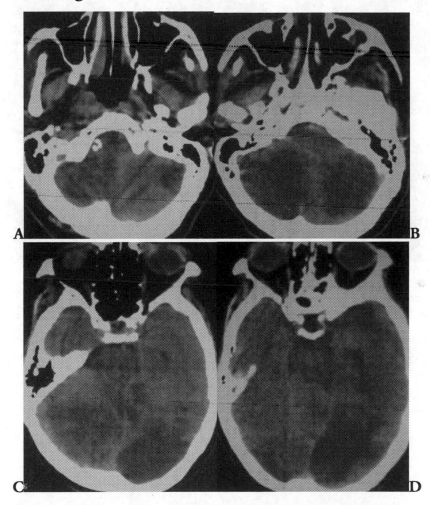

Plain brain CT Scan showing large low-attenuation areas involving both gray and white matter of the cerebellar hemispheres and occipital regions with obliteration of the cerebellar and occipital sulci and mass effect on the 4th ventricle. Note calcification of the right vertebral artery (image A).

Diagnosis: Vertebro-basilar Territory Infarction

Case 6

Clinical Presentation

A 63 year-old male patient, presented with right hemiparesis.

Radiological Findings

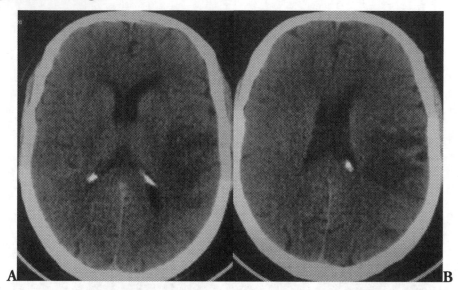

Nonenhanced brain CT Scan (A, B) demonstrates a large low-density area within the distribution of the superficial territory of the left middle cerebral artery (MCA) with loss of the gray-white matter differentiation and adjacent sulcal effacement. No significant ventricular compression or midline shift.

Diagnosis: Left MCA Infarction

Case 7

Clinical Presentation

A 57 year-old male patient fell while skiing 2 days ago and developed acute visual deterioration with left hemiplegia.

Radiological Findings

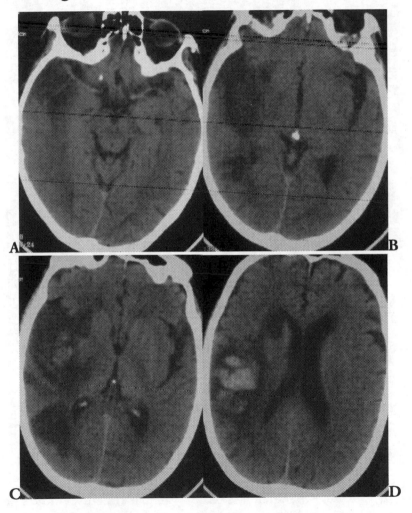

Plain CT Scan reveals a large low-attenuation area involving the right middle cerebral artery (MCA) territory with dense MCA, containing hyperdense areas (hemorrhagic transformation) with sulcal effacement and mild mass effect on the adjacent lateral ventricle.

Diagnosis: Hemorrhagic Transformation in Acute MCA Infarct

Case 8

Clinical Presentation

A 47 male patient with no particular past-history, presenting a sudden left hemiplegia.

Radiological Findings

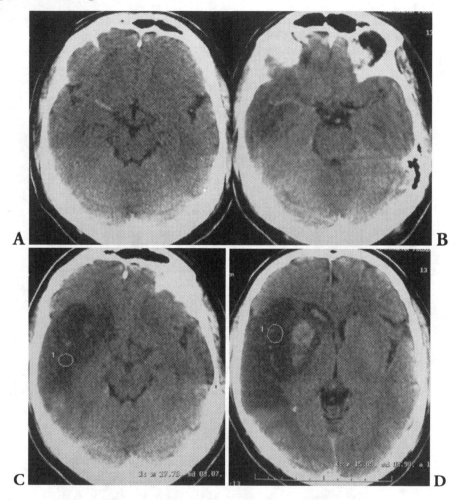

The first CT (A) shows a hyperattenuated linear vascular structure in the right temporal region (hyperdense MCA sign), representing thrombus formation within the vessel (early CT sign of ischemia). **The second CT (B, C, D)** done three days later shows a large low density area in the distribution of the MCA territory, containing hyperdense areas (hemorrhagic transformation of an ischemic infarct).

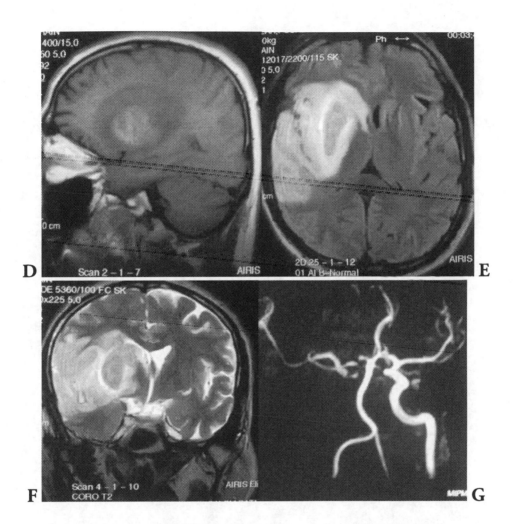

...continued, MR Scan (done four days later) sagittal T1 (D), axial FLAIR (E), coronal T2 (F) and MRA 3D-TOF (I) images show the extension of the infarct in the right MCA territory as a large area of low-T1 and high-T2 and FLAIR signal intensity, containing area of hemorrhage drawing the lentiform nucleus. The MRA shows complete thrombosis of the right internal carotid artery (ICA) and partial of M1 segment of MCA,which is supplied by the right anterior and posterior communicating arteries.

Diagnosis: Hemorrhagic Transformation of Right MCA Infarct with Complete Thrombosis of the ICA and Partially of M1-segment of the MCA

Case 9

Clinical Presentation

A 53 year-old male patient with acute onset of right hemiplegia.

Radiological Findings

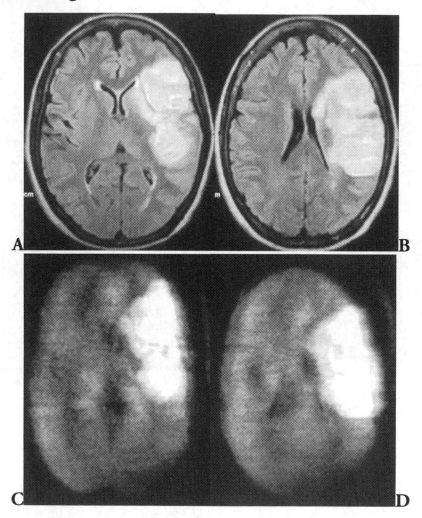

MRI Scan axial FLAIR (A, B) and DWI-EPI (C, D) showing a Large area of high-signal intensity in the distribution of the left middle cerebral artery territory with effacement of the adjacent cortical sulci and mild mass effect on the left lateral ventricle. The diffusion-weighted sequence demonstrates the ischemic region as an area of low diffusion or high signal intensity.

Diagnosis: Acute Left MCA Infarction

Case 10

Clinical Presentation

An 84 year-old hypertensive female patient presented with left upper arm crural paresis and frontal signs.

Radiological Findings

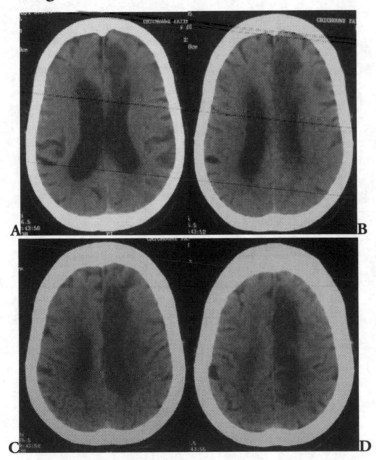

Plain brain CT Scan reveals a low attenuation abnormality involving the left frontal lobe in the distribution of the anterior cerebral artery territory (ACA). Mass effect is present on the adjacent lateral ventricle with effacement of the overlying cortical sulci.

Diagnosis: ACA Infarction

Case 11

Clinical Presentation

A 52 year-old male patient with Broca's aphasia and right monoparesis.

Radiological Findings

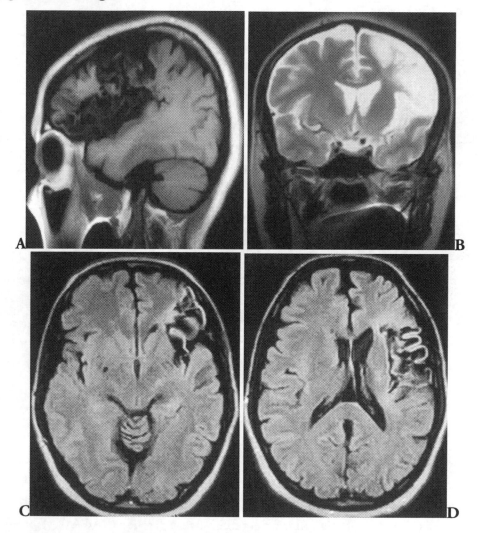

MR Scan, sagittal T1 (A), coronal T2 (B) and axial FLAIR (C, D) showing a large low-T1 and FLAIR and high T2 signal intensity area of the left fronto-insular region in the distribution of the superficial MCA territory with cortical atrophy, surrounded by a high signal area on FLAIR images indicating gliosis and demyelinisation. Note the dilatation of the ipsilateral LV and sylvian fissure indicating and old stroke.

Diagnosis: Old Infarction in MCA Territory

Case 12

Clinical Presentation

A 6 months old male child with history of neonatal neurological distress.

Radiological Findings

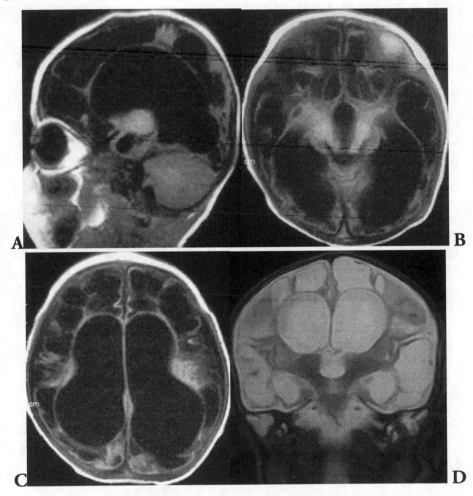

MR Scan sagittal (A) and axial (B, C) T1 and coronal T2-weighted images demonstrate a complete liquefaction of the cerebral hemispheres, which are replaced by large cysts of low-T1 and high-T2 signal intensity with thin septations and dilated ventricular system. Septae composed of glial cells and some viable neurons are seen as linear strands isointense to the brain tissue on both sequences. Note preservation of the cerebrum, which is considered as another typical findings.

Diagnosis: Diffuse Multicystic Encephalomalacia

Case 13

Clinical Presentation

A 9 year-old male child, presented with mental retardation and past-history of birth asphyxia.

Radiological Findings

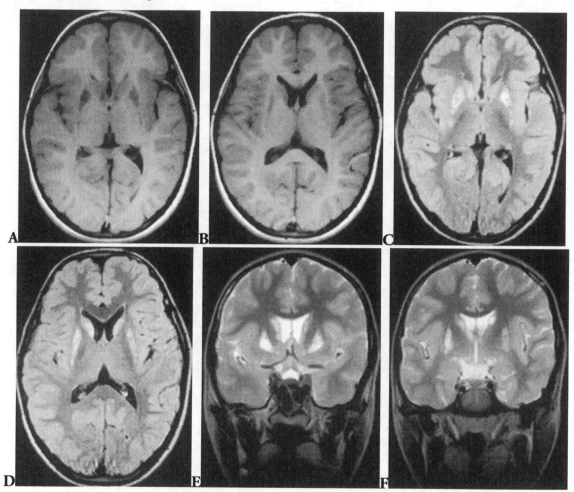

MR Scan, axial T1 (A, B), FLAIR (C, D) and coronal T2 (E, F) weighted images showing a bilateral and symmetrical low-T1 and high-T2 and FLAIR signal-intensity of the lenticular and caudate nuclei. No other brain abnormality.

Diagnosis: Sequelae of Neonatal Anoxic/Ischemic Encephalopathy

Case 14

Clinical Presentation

A 72 year-old hypertensive female patient brought to the emergency department with left sided hemplegia and altered level of consciousness.

Radiological Findings

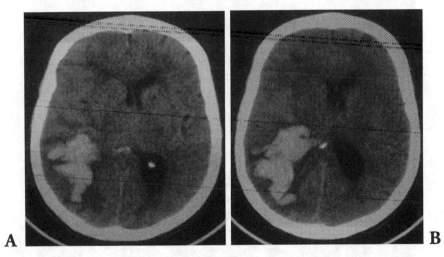

A   B

Nonenhanced brain CT Scan showing a large spontaneously hyperdense intraparenchymal lesion located in the right temporo-occipital region with surrounding hypodense edema, obliterating the adjacent ventricular horn with midline shift and sulcal effacement.

Diagnosis: Hemorrhagic Stroke

Case 15

Clinical Presentation

A 40 year-old male patient brought comatosed to the emergency department.

Radiological Findings

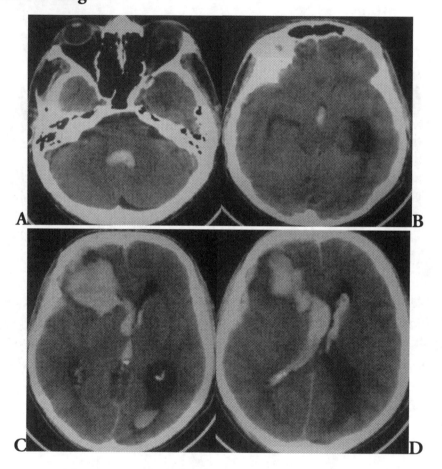

Plain brain CT Scan showing a large right frontal hematoma, surrounded by low-density area of edema with extensive intraventricular hemorrhage seen in the 4th, 3rd and lateral ventricles which are dilated with effacement of the cerebral sulci (due to cerebral edema) and midline shift to the left. There is a right fronto-temporal crescentic-shaped, homogeneous high-density collection of blood (subdural hematoma) due to a dissection of intraparenchymal hematoma into subarachnoid, then subdural space. No bone injury seen on the bone setting (not shown).

Diagnosis: Hemorrahgic CVA with Intra-ventricular Extension and SDH

Case 16

Clinical Presentation

A 25 year-old female with 10 days history of severe headache and diplopia.

Radiological Findings

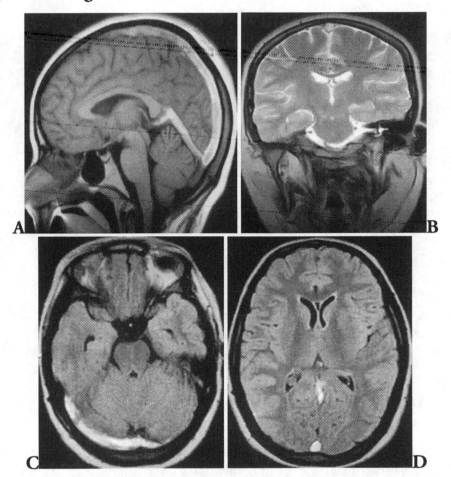

**Non-enhanced MR Scan sagittal T1 (A), coronal T2 (B), and axial FLAIR (C, D)
images** showing a hyperintense appearance in all sequences of the right lateral, straight
and superior sagittal sinuses indicating cerebral venous sinuses thrombosis. No venous
ischemic changes seen at both infra-or supra-tentorial level.

Diagnosis: Cerebral Venous Sinus Thrombosis (CVST)

Case 17

Clinical Presentation

A 23 year-old female patient with history of 6 months of headache without any neurological deficits.

Radiological Findings

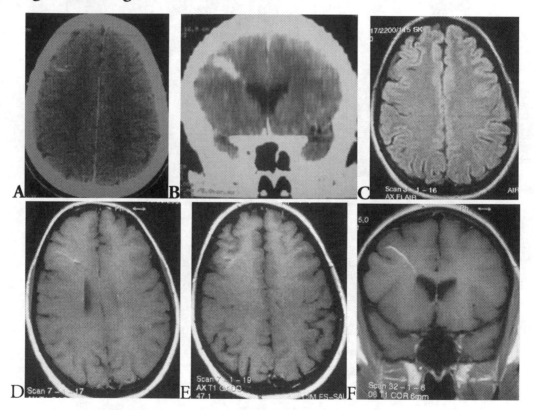

Postcontrast CT axial (A) with coronal reconstruction (B) and MR Scan axial FLAIR (C) and postcontrast axial (D, E) and coronal T1 images: The enhanced CT Scan shows a densely enhancing linear structure in the right frontal lobe, coursing between the frontal horn of the right lateral ventricle and the inner table of skull. The MR sequences show a linear signal void structure on FLAIR image intensely enhanced after gadolinium administration with medusa-like branching (image E).

Diagnosis: Cerebral Venous Angioma

Case 18

Clinical Presentation

A 39 year-old female patient, complaining of chronic headaches.

Radiological Findings

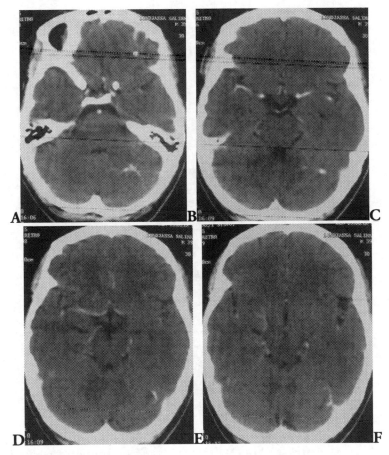

Enhanced brain CT Scan showing an enlarged enhanced left cerebellar vessel, giving a caput medusa shape appearance, converging to a draining vein than into the left lateral venous sinus. No surrounding edema or mass effect.

Diagnosis: Venous Angioma

Case 19

Clinical Presentation

A 26 year-old female patient with history of chronic headaches and generalized epilepsy.

Radiological Findings

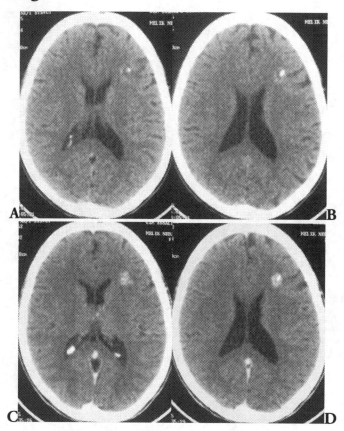

Pre-(A, B) and post-contrast (C, D) brain CT Scan showing a small left frontal hypodense lesion containing punctuate calcifications with significant enhancement after contrast administration. No surrounding edema or mass effect on the adjacent frontal horn.

Diagnosis: Cavernous Angioma

Case 20

Clinical Presentation

A 28 year-old female patient with history of generalized epilepsy.

Radiological Findings

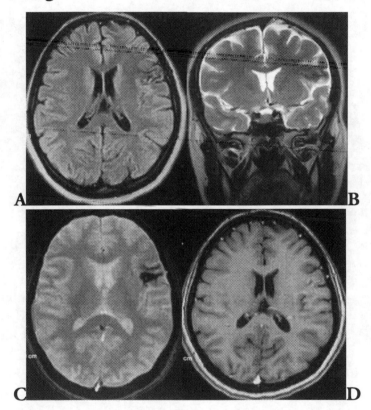

MR Scan, axial FLAIR (A), coronal T2 (B), axial T*2-GE (C) and post-contrast axial T2 (D) images reveal a small quadriangular lesion of left frontal cortico-subcortical location. This lesion appears slightly hypointense on FLAIR and T2, hypointense on T2-GE with central hyperintensity with no surrounding edema and no enhancement after gadolinium administration.

Diagnosis: Cavernous Angioma

Case 21

Clinical Presentation

A 31 year-old male patient with recent epilepsy.

Radiological Findings

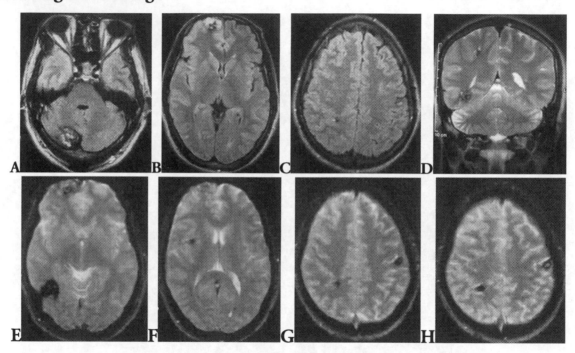

Brain MR, axial FLAIR (A, B, C), coronal T2 (D) and axial T*2-GE (E, F, G, H)-weighted images showing multiple lesions of cortical and sub-cortical location, one in the right cerebellum of heterogeneous signal centrally and hypointense peripherally, another similar lesion is seen in the right frontal lobe; the other lesions are mainly hypointense on T2-GE and located in the fronto=parietal regions.

Diagnosis: Multiple Cavernous Angiomas

Case 22

Clinical Presentation

A 72 year-old female patient known to have heart disease under sintron (acenocoumarol) tablets, presented with three days history of headaches, diplopia and convergent strabism.

Radiological Findings

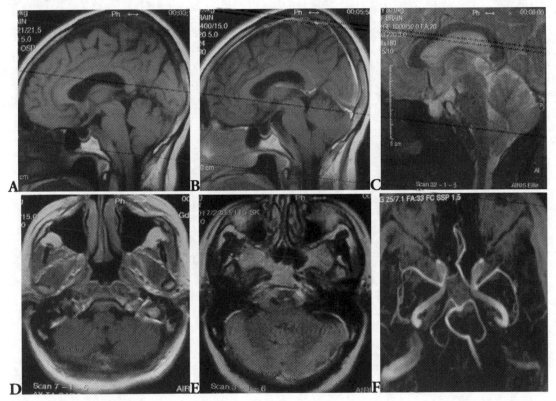

MR Scan, pre-and post-contrast sagittal (A, B), coronal GE-T*2 (C), post-contrast axial T1 (D), axial FLAIR (E) and MRA 3D-TOF (F) showing a pre-pontic and retro-clival fusiform mass of complex signal intensity, extending from the dorsum sellae to the foramen magnum. On T1 this mass shows a sediment of high signal with no enhancement after gadolinium administration. The MRA did not reveal any abnormality of the basilar or vertebral arteries.

Diagnosis : Spontaneous Retroclival Hematoma (in patient under anti-coagulant)

Case 23

Clinical Presentation

An 8 year-old female child with long history of seizures.

Radiological Findings

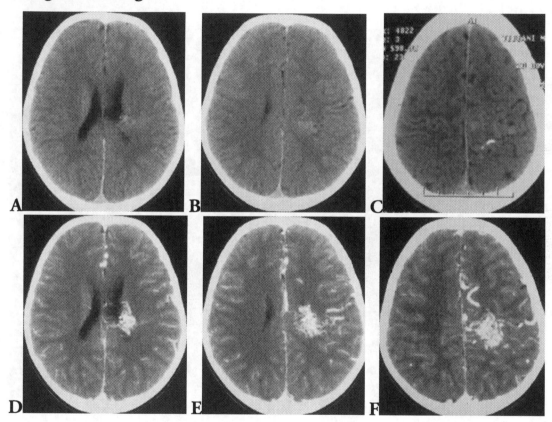

Pre-(A , B, C) and post-contrast (D, E, F) brain CT Scan showing left para-and juxta-ventricular isodense serpiginous structures, containing linear calcification with intense and synchronous enhancement to the normal vascular structures, representing the nidus of an arterio-venous malformation. Note dilated draining cortical veins drained into the superior sagittal sinus.

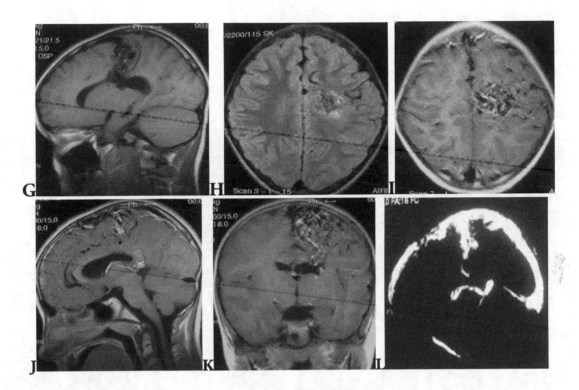

...**Continued, MR Scan, pre-contrast sagittal T1 (G), axial FLAIR (H), post-contrast axial (I), sagittal (J) and coronal (K) T1-weighted images with MRV-2D-TOF (L)** demonstrate a tangle of serpiginous flow void structures with areas of high signal (slower flow), extending to the body of the corpus callosum and left lateral ventricle. The MRV shows the dilated draining cortical veins, drained into the superior sagittal sinus.

Diagnosis: Arterio-venous Malformation (AVM)

Case 24

Clinical Presentation

An 81 year-old female patient with history of chronic headaches, presented with right 3rd nerve palsy.

Radiological Findings

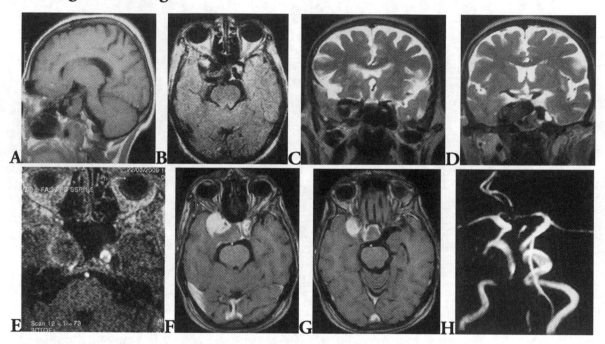

MR Scan, sagittal T1 (A), axial FLAIR (B), coronal T2 (C, D), Axial native 3D-TOF (E), post-contrast axial T1 (F, G) and MRA-3D-TOF (H) images showing a saccular structure filling the left cavernous sinus with supra-sellar extension with two components, the first component shows a signal void on T1, T2 and FLAIR with intense and synchronous enhancement to the left internal carotid artery; the second component is mainly of supra-sellar location, compressing certainly the right 3rd nerve and appears isointense on T1 and FLAIR and hypointense on T2 with no enhancement after contrast administration. On MRA-3D-TOF the right intra-cavernous and supra-clinoid portion of the internal carotid artery (ICA) shows reduced caliber, indicating partial thrombosis.

Diagnosis: Partially Thrombosed Aneurysm Of Intra-cavernous and Supra-clinoid ICA

Case 25

Clinical Presentation

A 40 year-old male patient, complaining of isolated headaches.

Radiological Findings

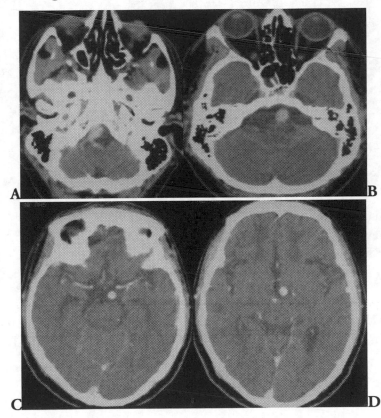

Enhanced brain CT Scan demonstrates a moderate fusiform dilatation of the basiar artery extending just above the vertebral arteries (as shown on image A).up to the 3rd ventricle level

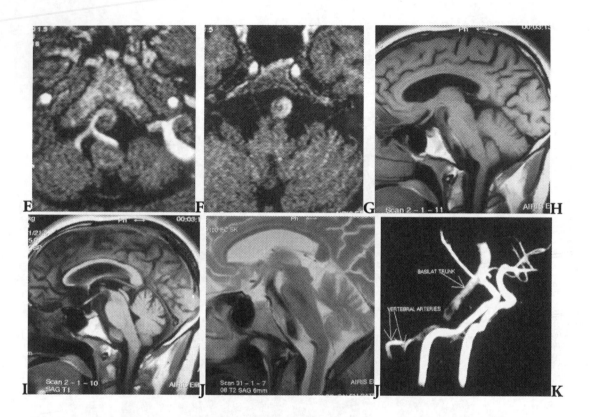

...Continued, MR Scan, 3D-TOF native axial images (E, F), nonenhanced sagittal T1 (G, I), sagittal T2 (J) and MRA 3D-TOF (K) images show a moderately dilated basilar artery, partially thrombosed in its inferior portion as shown on the native 3D-TOF, sagittal T1 and T2 images. The MRA confirms the fusifom dilatation and partial thrombosis.

Diagnosis: Partially thrombosed Basilar Artery Aneurysm

Case 26

Clinical Presentation

A 5 months old female child with history of CHF and repeated tonico-clonic seizures.

Radiological Findings

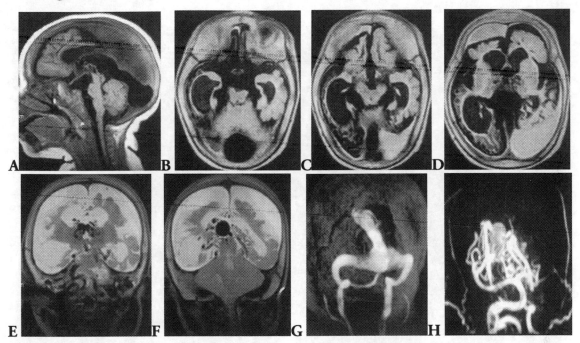

MR Scan, sagittal T1 (A), axial FLAIR (B, C, D), coronal T2 (E, F), MRV-2D-TOF (G) and MRA-3D-TOF (H) images reveal a large flow-void demarcated vascular structure, posterior to the 3rd ventricle corresponding to a vein of Galen malformation with dilated draining venous system and trocular. The MRA shows the mural type of Galen varix with enlarged middle artery branches and multiple thalamoperforater feeders terminating in the varix. Note some cerebellar and cerebral atrophy mainly of the right hemisphere with right frontal and left occipital chronic subdural hematomas.

Diagnosis: Vein of Galen Aneurysm with Damaged Brain

Case 27

Clinical Presentation

A 71 year-old diabetic and hypertensive male patient with three weeks history of Mnesic disorder and lipothymia.

Radiological Findings

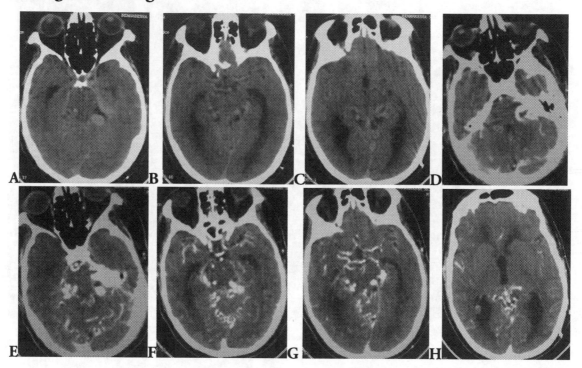

Pre-(A, B, C) and post-contrast (D, E, F, G, H) brain CT Scan: Note extensive evidence of dilated spontaneously hyperintense dilated venous structures, enhancing after contrast administration, visible around the brainstem and basal cisterns, drained into the straight sinus. The diffuse nature of enlarged deep and superficial venous system implies venous hypertension. Note dilated 3rd and lateral ventricles.

Diagnosis: Dural Arteriovenous Malformation (DAVM)

Case 28

Clinical Presentation

A 42 year-old patient involved in road traffic accident.

Radiological Findings

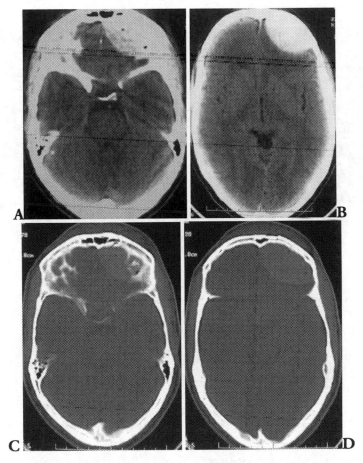

Brain CT Scan with bone settings demonstrates a large homogeneous hyperdense lens-shaped (biconvex) epidural hematoma, containing air-bubbles (localized pneumocephalus), located in the frontal region with obliteration of the adjacent frontal horn and associated extracranial soft tissue swelling. The extra-axial location of the hematoma is evidenced by a broad-base area of contact with skull, sharply defined interface with the brain, and complete absence of parenchyma within the lesion. Bone setting shows complex fracture of the frontal sinus wall.

Diagnosis: Epidural Hematoma

Case 29

Clinical Presentation

A 16 year-old male victim of a brutal attack, received numerous kicks to his head while lying on the ground and finally was hit by a big stone.

Radiological Findings

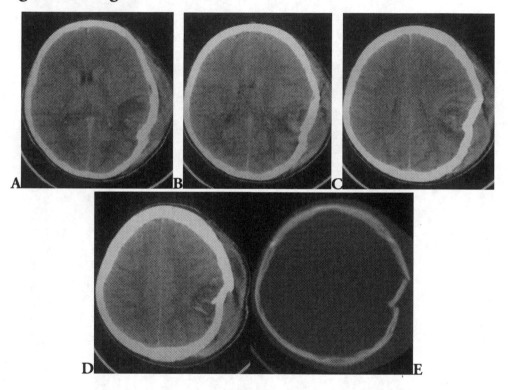

Plain brain CT Scan showing a large temporo-parietal low-density area containing high-density zones of hemorrhage with mass effect on the left lateral ventricle, depressed skull vault fracture and scalp hematoma.

Diagnosis: Edemato-hemorrhagic Contusion with Depressed Skull Fracture and Scalp Hematoma

Case 30

Clinical Presentation

A 50 year-old male patient, presented with frontal syndrome and left hemiparesis.

Radiological Findings

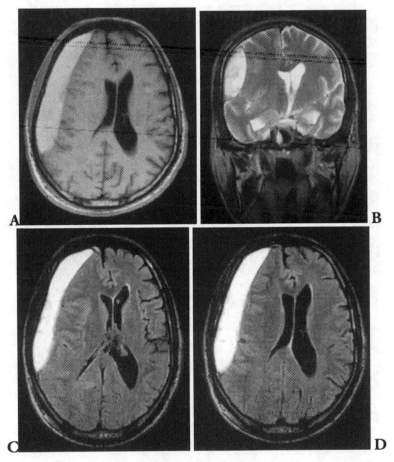

MR Scan, axial T1 (A), coronal T2 (B), axial FLAIR (C, D) images reveal a large right sided crescent-shaped subdural collection of high-T1, T2 and FLAIR signal intensity, interposed between the skull and compressed cerebral cortex. Numerous thin fibrous septations are noted within the hematoma on T2-weighted image, suggesting multiple compartments to the lesion. There is mass effect on the midline structures, obliterating partially the adjacent right LV with mild dilatation of the contra-lateral LV.

Diagnosis: Subacute Subdural Hematoma

Case 31

Clinical Presentation

A 72 year-old female patient with history of headaches and vertigo.

Radiological Findings

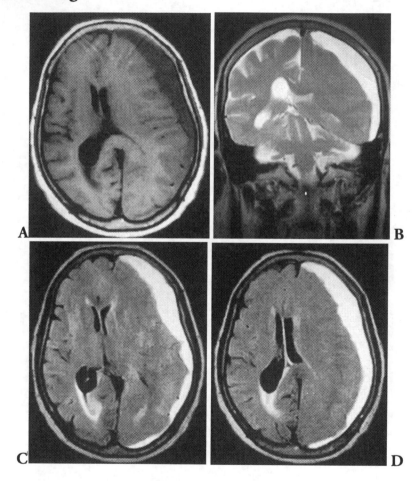

MR Scan, axial T1 (A), coronal T2 (B), axial FLAIR (C, D) images demonstrate a large left sided crescent-shaped subdural collection of low-T1 and high-T2 and FLAIR signal intensity, extending over the whole hemisphere, compressing the adjacent cerebral parenchyma, obliterating the left LV with mass effect on the midline structures and subfalcine herniation. The right lateral ventricle is dilated mainly is its posterior portion with interstitial peri-ventricular edema.

Diagnosis: Chronic Subdural Hematoma

Case 32

Clinical Presentation

A 30 year-old epileptic female with history of head traumatism (fell down after epileptic seizures).

Radiological Findings

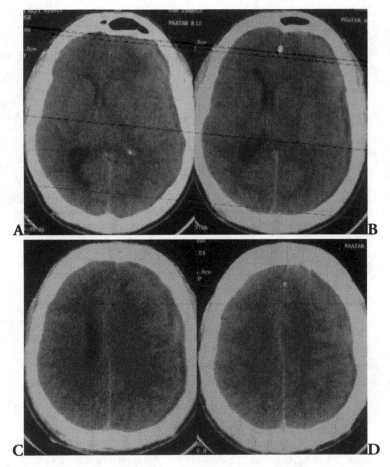

Plain brain CT Scan showing a left crescent shape fluid collection, interposed between the skull and compressed cerebral cortex with tapered margins and spread along the calvarium indicating its subdural location. This collection appears hypodense with localized hyperdense areas strongly suggestive of rebleed within chronic SDH. There is stricking mass effect with midline displacement (subfalcine herniation), compression of the ipsilateral lateral ventricle.

Diagnosis: Chronic SDH with Recent Rebleed

Case 33

Clinical Presentation

A 5 months old male child with increased head circumference.

Radiological Findings

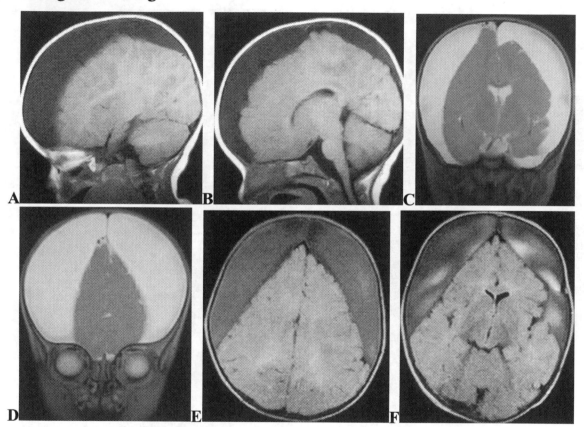

MR Scan, sagittal T1 (A, B), coronal T2 (C, D), and axial FLAIR (E,F) images showing a large bilateral subdural fluid collection of CSF signal intensity, mainly in the fronto-temporo-parietal regions, displacing the brain tissue inwards, and compressing symmetrically the ventricular system with no midline shift.

Diagnosis: Bilateral Subdural Hygroma

Case 34

Clinical Presentation

A 8 year-old male child presenting a recurrent pneumococcal meningitis with rhiorrhea., In his past-history with note a brain injury 2 years ago.

Radiological Findings

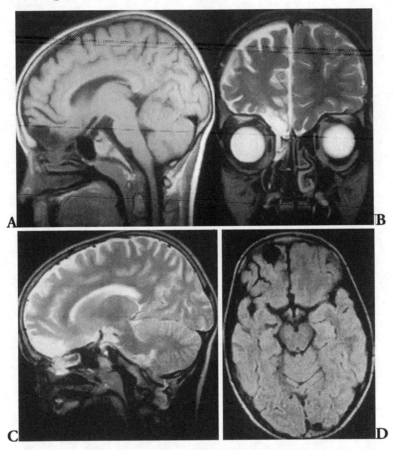

MR Scan, sagittal T1 (A), coronal and sagittal T2 (B, C) and axial FLAIR (D)-weighted images showing a right basi-frontal fluid collection identical to the CSF, in continuity with and other similar collection of the right anterior ethmoid region through an osseous defect of the roof of the ethmoid labyrinth. Otherwise, we note a reduced volume of the right cerebral hemisphere with enlarged cerebral suci (brain atrophy).

Diagnosis: Posttraumatic Osteo-dural Fistula

Infection and
Inflammatory Diseases

Case 35

Clinical Presentation

A 26 year-old female patient with history of fever and headache for several days with onset of seizures.

Radiological Findings

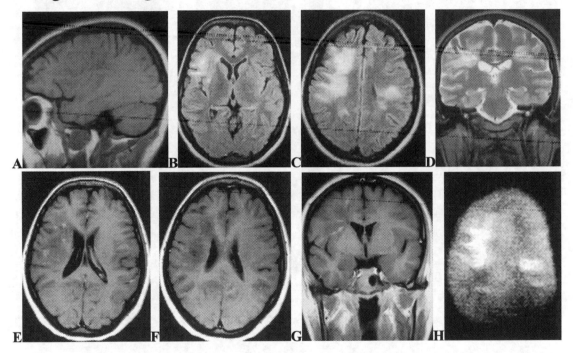

MR Scan, pre-contrast sagittal T1 (A), axial FLAIR (B, C), coronal T2 (D), post-contrast axial and coronal T1 (E, F, G) and DWI-EPI-PG (H) images show ill-defined low-T1 and high-T2 and FLAIR signal intensity areas involving the cortico-subcortical regions, right insular cortex and para-ventricular white matter mainly of the frontal lobes with focal areas of linear and nodular enhancement after gadolinium administration. The Diffusion echoplanar image shows prolonged diffusion (high signal) in these areas. The putamen are spared.

Diagnosis: Herpes Encephalitis

Case 36

Clinical Presentation

A 7 year-old male child with fever; confusional state and epilepsy.

Radiological Findings

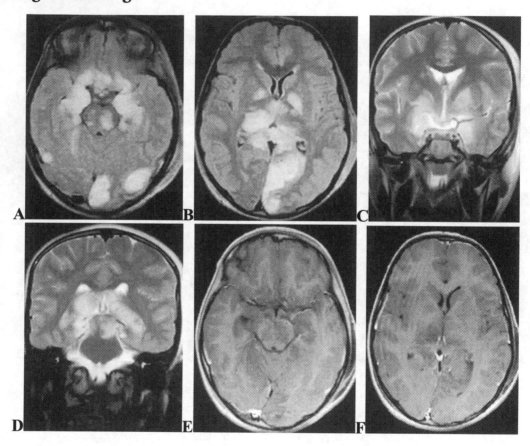

MR Scan, axial FLAIR (A, B), coronal T2 (C, D) and post-contrast axial T1 (E, F) weighted images demonstrate multiple low-T1 and high-FLAIR and T2 signal intensity areas with no enhancement after gadolinium administration, involving the brainstem, temporal lobes (mainly the hippocampi and unci), basi-frontal regions, basal ganglia, splenium, and occipital lobes mainly on the left. Obliteration of the temporal horns because of swelling of the hippocampi. Note that the putamen are spared.

Diagnosis: Multifocal Herpes Encephalitis

Case 37

Clinical Presentation

A 56 year-old man, with history of chronic discharge from the right ear, presented with severe headaches and vomiting for the last week with two attacks of drowsiness and difficulty in walking in the last two days.

Radiological Findings

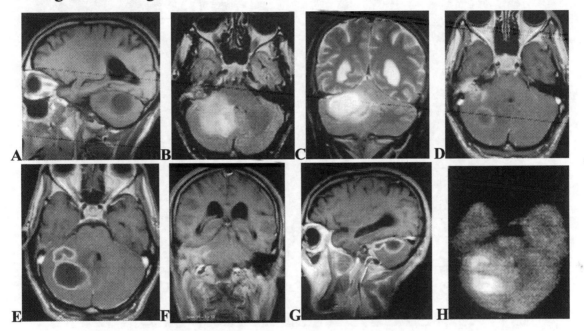

MR Scan, pre-contrast sagittal (A), axial FLAIR (B), coronal T2 (C), post-contrast axial (D, E), coronal (F) and sagittal (G), and DWI-EPI (H) images reveal a biloculated low-T1 and high-FLAIR and T2 right cerebellar lesion with thin and smooth ring-like enhancement, surrounded by area of vasogenic edema. The DWI image shows restricted diffusion (high signal). There is mass effect on the 4th ventricle, which is compressed and displaced to the left side with raised intraventriculat pressure (3rd & LV). Note the hyperintense filling on FLAIR image of the right middle ear and mastoid air-cells with enhancement on T1 images after gadolinium administration, representing an otomastoiditis.

Diagnosis: Cerebellar Abscess Complicating a Chronic Otomastoiditis

Case 38

Clinical Presentation

A 54 year-old female patient with history of fever and severe headaches.

Radiological Findings

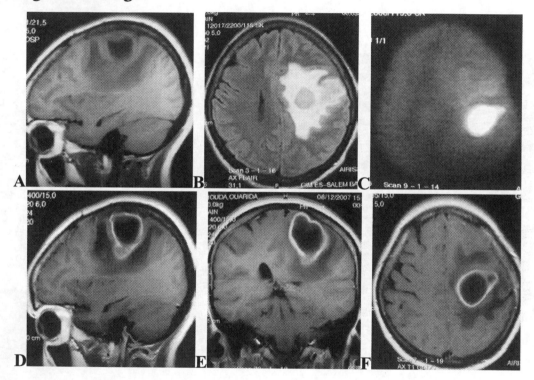

Brain MR Scan Pre-contrast sagittal (A), post-contrast sagittal (D), coronal (E), axial (F) T1 sequences, axial FLAIR (B) and EPI-DWI-TRS-PG (C) showing a large lobulated low-T1 and FLAIR lesion with thin and smooth ring-like enhancement, located in the left pre-central frontal lobe with large perilesional edema of low-T1 and high FLAIR signal intensity, obliterating partially the adjacent lateral ventricle with sulcal effacement. The diffusion weighted imaging (DWI) sequence shows restricted diffusion, excluding the possibility of brain tumor.

Diagnosis: Brain Abscess

Case 39

Clinical Presentation

A 30 year-old male patient with progressive headache, fever, and fainting.

Radiological Findings

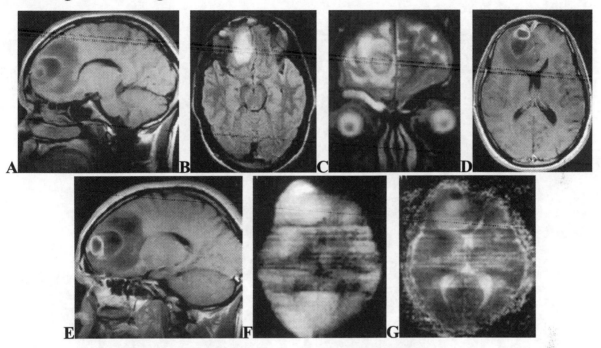

MR Scan, pre-contrast sagittal T1 (A), axial FLAIR (B), coronal T2 (C), post-contrast axial (D), sagittal (E)-T1, and DWI-EPI-PG (F) with ADC (G) images demonstrate a bi-loculated left frontal intra-axial lesion of low-T1 and high FLAIR and T2 signal intensity with a peripheral capsule which appears isointense on T1 and hypointense on T2 with ring like enhancement after gadolinium administration. The DWI image shows restricted diffusion (hypersignal) with decreased ADC. There is a significant edema around the lesion, obliterating the adjacent frontal horn. Note that the mucosal thickening of the frontal sinuses mainly on the left (sinusitis) adjacent to the frontal lesion.

Diagnosis: Brain abscess (caused by extension of frontal sinusitis)

Case 40

Clinical Presentation

A 17 year-old male patient, presenting headaches and fever. He was operated three weeks ago for a posttraumatic right temporal epidural hematoma.

Radiological Findings

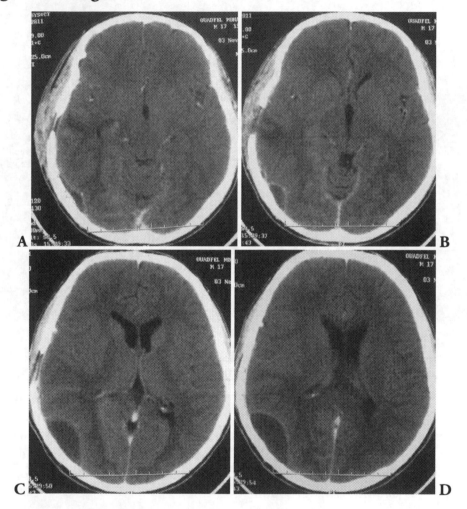

Enhanced brain CT Scan showing a right occipital extradural hypodense collection with thin rim of enhancement, obliterating the adjacent occipital horn. Note edematous hypodense area of the right temporal lobe adjacent to the craniotomy with swelling of the scalp soft tissue (post-operative changes).

Diagnosis: Extradural Empyema

Case 41

Clinical Presentation

A 9 year-old male child with history of repeated vomiting and headaches. On examination the patient had bilateral papilledema.

Radiological Findings

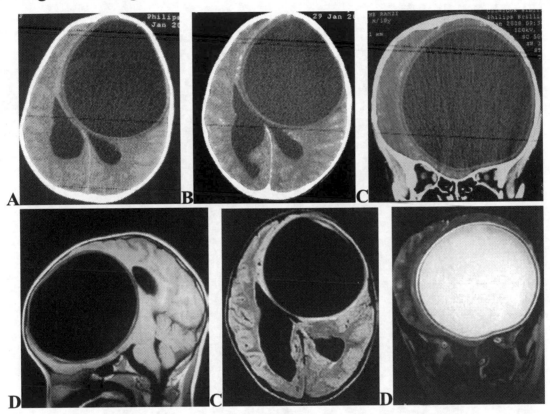

Pre (A)-and post-contrast (B, C) brain CT Scan, and MR Scan: unenhanced sagittal T1 (D), axial FLAIR (C), and coronal T2 (D): The CT shows a large, ovoid well-defined left frontal cystic lesion with thin and regular internal membrane isodense to the cortical gray matter, not enhanced by contrast administration and with no peri-lesional edema, obliterating the 3rd ventricle and anterior portion of the lateral ventricles with dilated posterior portion. Note an important mass effect on the midline structures. The MR sequences shows the same findings with low-T1 and FLAIR and high-T2 of the cystic lesion, the internal membrane appears hypointense on all sequences.

Diagnosis: Cerebral Hydatid Cyst

Case 42

Clinical Presentation

A 6 year-old male child with 4 days history of headaches, fever with irritabilty. 10 days prior, this child had symptoms of upper respiratory infection. CSF study reveals mild leucocytosis with predominantly lymphocytes and no organisms.

Radiological Findings

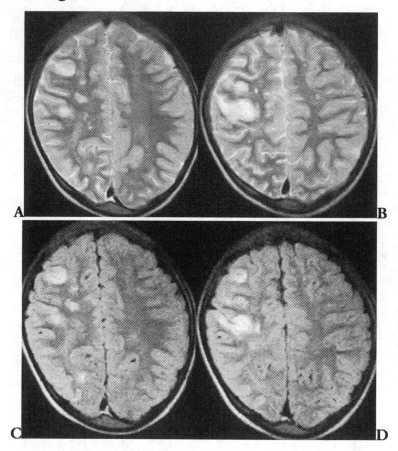

MRI Scan axial T2-weighted images (A, B) and FLAIR (C, D) reveal Multiple scattered areas of high T2 and FLAIR signal intensity, located at the gray-white matter junction of the right frontal and parietal lobes, and centrum semi-ovale.

Diagnosis: ADEM (Acute Demyelinating Encephalomyelitis)

Case 43

Clinical Presentation

A 28 year-old female patient with history of fatigability, altered personality, and focal neurological complaints.

Radiological Findings

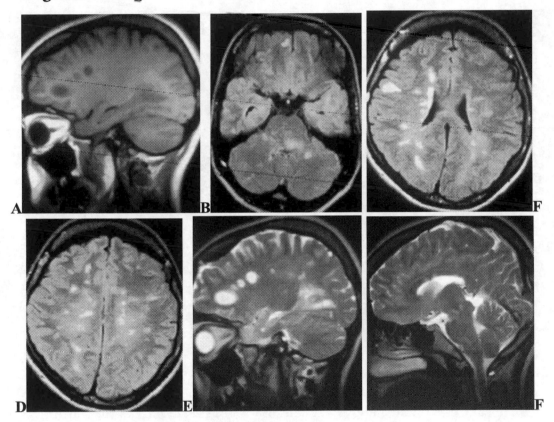

MRI Scan pre-contrast sagittal T1 (A), axial FLAIR (B, C, D) and coronal T2 (E, F)-weighted images showing multiple low-T1 and high-FLAIR and T2WI ovoid lesions of various size are seen in the brainstem, white matter of the cerebellar and cerebral hemispheres, several of which are callosal-septal on sagittal T2WI and periventricular oriented perpendicular to the lateral ventriclar surface. Non enhancement of the lesions seen on fat-suppressed postcontrast T1WI.(not shown).

Diagnosis: Multiple Sclerosis (MS)

Case 44

Clinical Presentation

A 39 year-old female patient with no particular past-history, presented with a pyramidal syndrome of the right hemi-body and left upper limb..

Radiological Findings

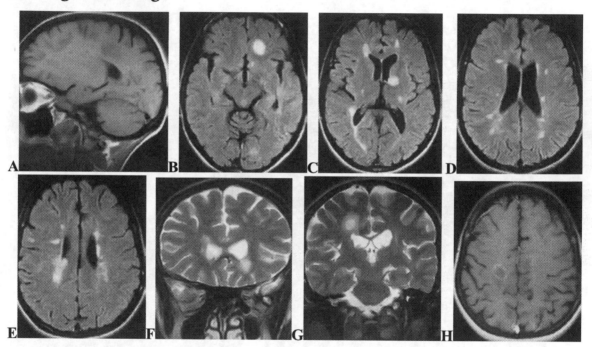

MRI Scan pre-contrast sagittal T1 (A), axial FLAIR (B, C, D, E) and coronal T2 (F, G) and post-contrast axial T1 (H) weighted images showing numerous low-T1 and high-FLAIR and T2 round and ovoid lesions of various size, located in the subcortical and peri-ventricular white matter and in the centrum semi-ovale. Some of them are oriented perpendicular to the lateral ventriclar surface. The largest lesions are located in the deep left frontal white matter, left internal capsule and centrum semi-ovale, the latest one shows peripheral ring enhancement after gadolinium administration (image H), indicating active plaque. Note mild enlargement of the cerebral sulci with subtle dilatation of the ventricular system indicating brain atrophy.

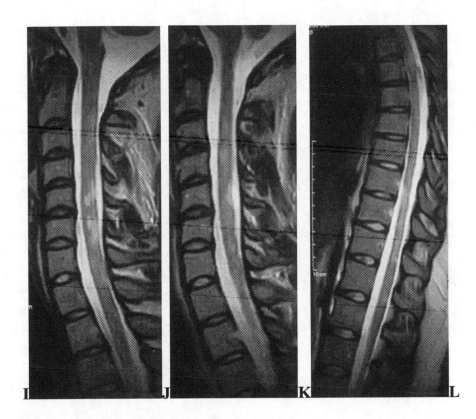

I   J   K   L

…Continued, MR Scan sagittal T2-weighted images of the cervical (I, J) and dorsal (L) spinal cord reveal a mild swelling of the cervical spinal cord with multiple intra-medullary high-signal lesions of various size, extending from the bulbo-medullary junction up to the conus medullaris

Diagnosis: Cerebro-Medullary Multiple Sclerosis with Active Plaque

Degenerative Diseases

Case 45

Clinical Presentation

A 21 year-old female patient presented with cerebellar ataxia.

Radiological Findings

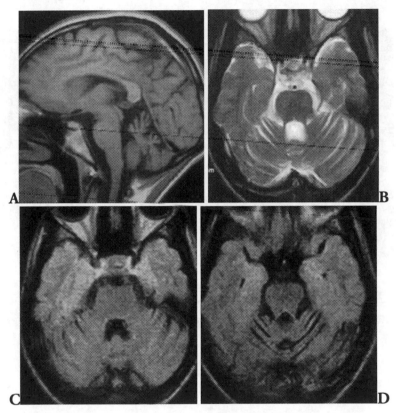

MR Scan sagittal T1 (A), axial T2 (B), and FLAIR (C, D) showing an enlargement of the cerebello-vermian sulci and peri-cerebellar CSF spaces with dilated 4th ventricle.

Diagnosis: Cerebellar atrophy

Case 46

Clinical Presentation

A 86 year-old male patient with history of progressive impairment of memory and intellectual function.

Radiological Findings

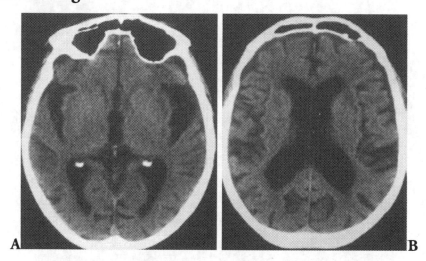

Plain brain CT Scan (A, B) reveals a diffuse enlargement of the cerebral sulci and sylvian fissures with proportional dilatation of the ventricular system. No cerebral focal lesion seen.

Diagnosis: Cerebral Atrophy

Neoplasms

Case 47

Clinical Presentation

A 5 year-old female child, presented with left hemiparesis and right 4th nerve palsy.

Radiological Findings

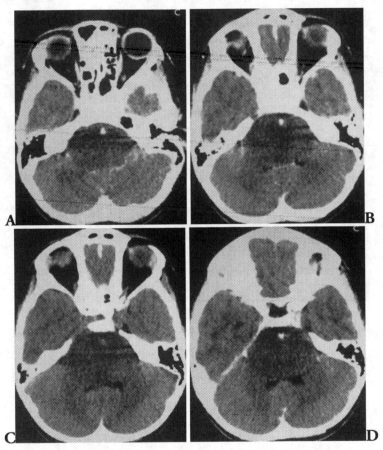

Enhanced brain CT Scan showing a large non-enhanced hypodense mass enlarging the brainstem, filling the posterior fossa cisterns, encircling the lower portion of the basilar artery and obliterating the floor of the 4th ventricle.

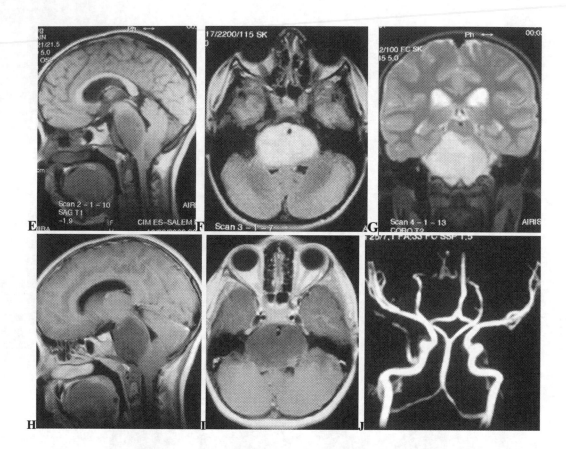

...Continued, MR Scan pre-contrast sagittal T1 (E), axial FLAIR (F), coronal T2 (G), post-contrast sagittal (H) and axial (I) T1-weighted images and MRA (J) show that the previously described brainstem lesion appears hypointense on T1, hyperintense on FLAIR and T2 with no enhancement after gadolinium administration, encircling the distal portion of the vertebral arteries and proximal basilar artery as shown on the axial images and MRA. Note the tonsilar heriation in the foramen magnum with hydrosyringomyelia of the cervical spinal cord indicating Chiari I malformation.

Diagnosis: Brainstem Glioma in Child with Chiari I Malformation

Case 48

Clinical presentation

A 10 year-old male child with history of irritability and vomiting.

Radiological Findings

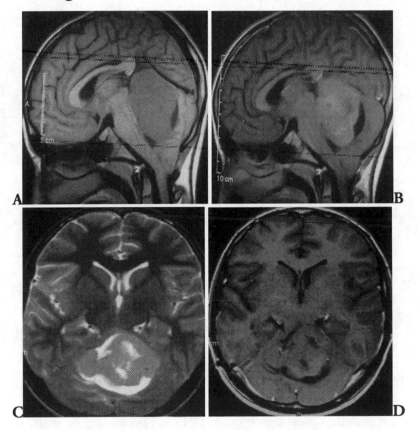

Pre-and post-gadolinium sagittal (A, B) and axial (D)T1-weighted, and axial T2 (C) weighted images showing a large, lobulated 4th ventricular tumoral mass, slightly hypointense on T1 and isointense to the gray matter on T2-weighted, containing necrotic areas which appear hypointense on T1 and hyperintense on T2. After gadolinium administration the tumor shows moderate and inhomogeneous enhancement. The brainstem is compressed and displaced anteriorly, the cerebellar parenchyma posteriorly with tonsilar herniation through the foramen magnum, upward displacement of the straight sinus with mass effect on the splenium of the corpus callosum. Note that right ventricular shunt (image D) has significantly reduced the intra-ventricular pressure.

Diagnosis: Ependymoma of the 4th ventricle

Case 49

Clinical Presentation

A 10 year-old male child presented with signs of increased intracranial pressure.

Radiological Findings

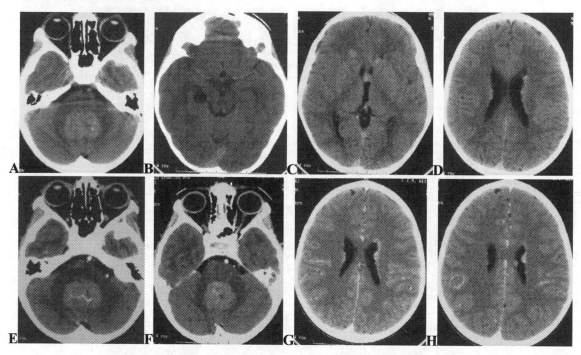

Pre-(A, B, C, D) and post-contrast (E, F, G, H) brain CT Scan showing a large median mass of the posterior fossa apparently located within the 4th ventricle, mildly hyperdense, containing punctiform calcification with mild and heterogeneous enhancement after contrast administration, compressing the brainstem with mild obstructive hydrocephalus. Note a small cystic lesion in the right medial temporal fossa (image B) corresponding to an arachnoid cyst of the choroid fissure. Presence of multiple subependymal nodular masses isodense to the cortical gray matter lining the lateral ventricles and frontal horns (subependymal heterotopias of gray matter).

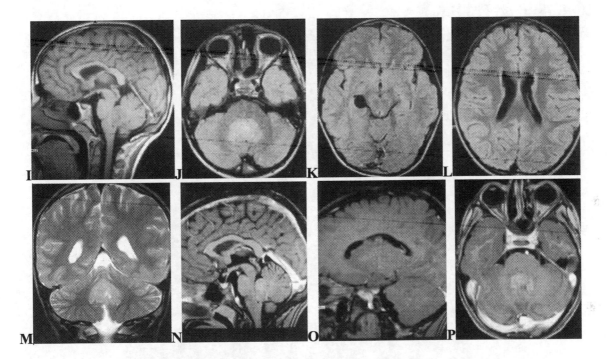

...Continued, pre-contrast sagittal T1 (I), axial FLAIR (J, K, L), coronal T2 (M) and post-contrast sagittal (N, O) and axial (P) T1-weighted images confirm that the lesion of the posterior cerebral fossa is located within the 4th ventricle and appears isointense to the gray matter on T1 and T2 and hyperintense on FLAIR with moderate and heterogeneous enhancement after gadolinium administration. Here the subependymal heterotopia is well-visualized as multiple small sybependymal nodules isointense to the gray matter on all sequences lining the wall of the lateral ventricles. Also the small arachnoid cyst of the choroid fissure is well-visualized in the right medial temporal fossa.

Diagnosis: Ependymoma of 4th Ventricle with Subependymal Heterotopia of Gray Matter and Arachnoid Cyst of Choroid Fissure

Case 50

Clinical Presentation

A 56 female patient with past-history of breast Ca, presenting a pyramidal syndrome of the four limbs, posterior cordonal syndrome and static cerebellar syndrome.

Radiological Findings

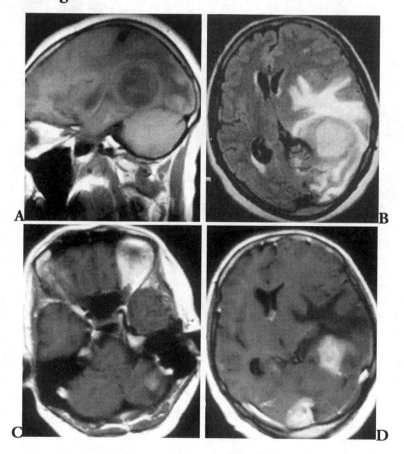

MRI Scan, pre-contrast sagittal (A),post-contrast axial (C,D) T1 and axial T2 (B)-weighted images There are at least three enhancing lesions, two infra-tentorial and one supra-tentorial of left temporo-occipital location which appears hypointense on T1 and hyperintense on T2 with large area of perilesional vasogenic edema, compressing the adjacent ventricular system with midline shift.

Diagnosis: Brain Metastases

Case 51

Clinical Presentation

An 82 year-old male patient with past-history of laryngeal Ca, presented with left hemiparesis, mainly of the upper limb.

Radiological Findings

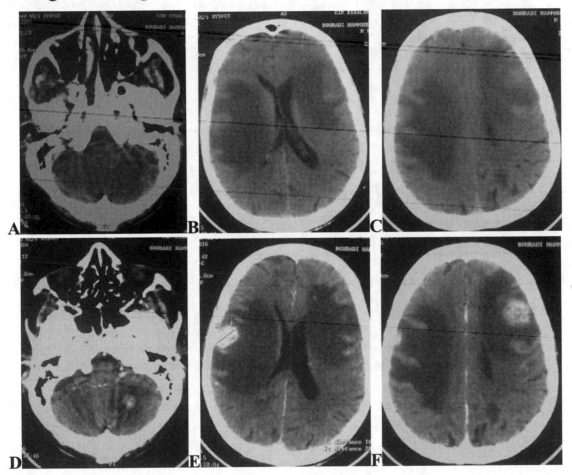

Pre-(A, B, C) and post-contrast (D, E, F) CT Scan images show three isodense lesions with nodular enhancement, one located in the left cerebellar hemisphere with surrounding vasogenic edema, obliterating partially the 4th ventricle; the two others are located in the frontal regions at the white-gray matter junction with significant surrounding vasogenic edema, sulcal effacement and mass effect on the lateral ventricles.

Diagnosis: Brain Metastases (from Laryngeal Ca.)

Case 52

Clinical Presentation

A 34 year-old patient, presented with bilateral papilledema.

Radiological Findings

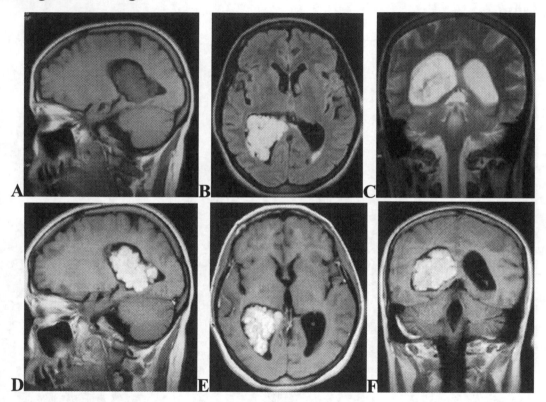

MR Scan, sagittal pre(A)-and post-contrast (D), post-contrast axial (E), coronal (F) T1, axial FLAIR (B) and coronal T2 (C)-weighted sequences reveal a large low-T1 and high-T2 and FLAIR, lobulated mass enlarging the trigone of the right lateral ventricle with small central vascular flow voids, intensely enhanced by contrast administration with no surrounding vasogenic edema or invasion of the adjacent cerebral parenchyma. Note that the left trigone is also dilated.

Diagnosis: Choroid Plexus Papilloma

Case 53

Clinical Presentation

A 37 year-old male patient presented with signs of increase intra-cranial pressure.

Radiological Findings

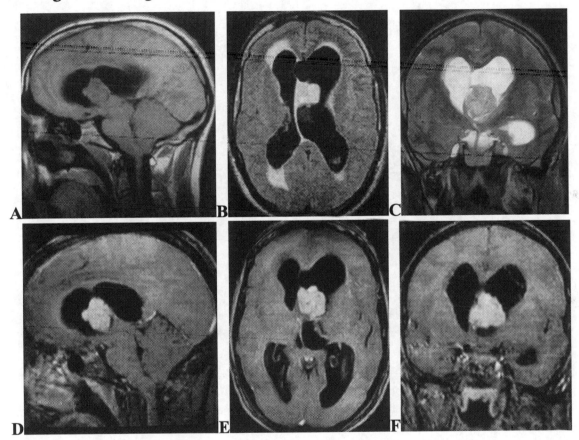

MR Scan pre-contrast sagittal T1 (A), axial FLAIR (B), coronal T2 (C) and post-contrast sagittal (D), axial (E) and coronal (F) T1-weighted images demonstrate an intra-ventricular lobulated mass, attached to the interventricular septum and bulging into the left lateral ventricle. It appears isointense on T1 and T2 and hyperintense on FLAIR with intense and homogeneous enhancement after gadolinium administration, obstructing the foramina of Monro with dilated lateral ventricles and peri-ventricular interstitial edema (due to trans-ependymal resorption of CSF).

Diagnosis: Choroid Plexus Lateral Ventricular Papilloma with Hydrocephalus

Case 54

Clinical Presentation

A 7 year-old female child with history of headaches and intermittent vomiting.

Radiological Findings

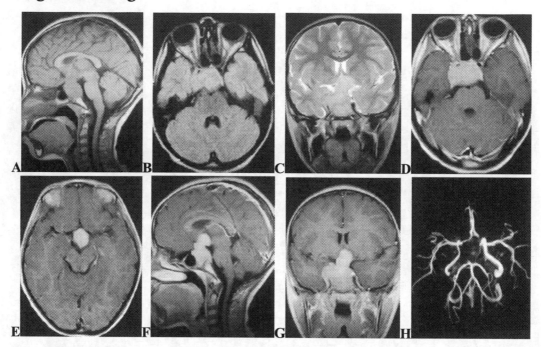

Brain MR, pre-contrast sagittal T1 (A), axial FLAIR (B), coronal T2 (C) and post-contrast axial (D, E), sagittal (F), and coronal (G), with MRA-3D-TOF (H) showing a bilobulated intra-and supra-sellar mass, slightly hypointense on T1, isointense on FLAIR and T2 with intense and homogeneous enhancement after contrast administration. This mass fills the opto-chiasmatic cistern and compresses the optic chiasma superiorly, fills the sellar region and compresses the pituitary gland inferiorly. Laterally this mass fills the right cavernous sinus and reduces the caliber of the internal carotid artery as seen on the MRA image. Note also a mild retro-clival extension filling partially the pre-pontic cistern.

Diagnosis: Germinoma

Case 55

Clinical Presentation

A 25 year-old male patient with persistent headaches and vomiting.

Radiological Findings

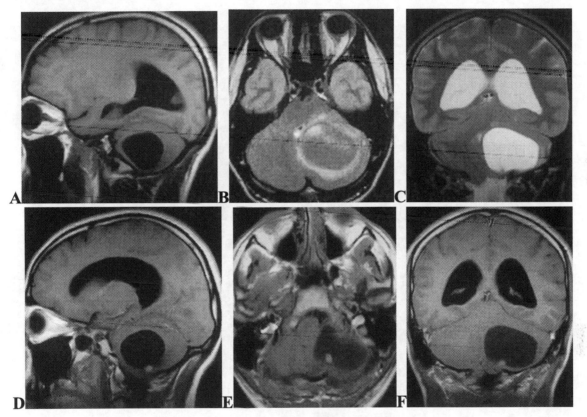

MR Scan, pre-contrast sagittal T1 (A), axial FLAIR (B), coronal T2 (C), post-contrast sagittal (D), axial (E) and coronal (F) T1-weighted images demonstrate a large left cerebellar cystic mass, hypointense on T1, isointense on FLAIR and hyperintense on T2 with thin rim of peripheral vasogenic edema. After gadolinium administration there is a small rounded enhancing mural nodule of postero-inferior location. There is mass effect on the brainstem and the 4th ventricle which is compressed and displaced to the right with dilated 3rd and lateral ventricles (tri-ventricular hydrocephalus).

Diagnosis: Cerebellar Hemangioblastoma

Case 56

Clinical Presentation

A 19 year-old female patient presented with signs of raised intracranial pressure.

Radiological Findings

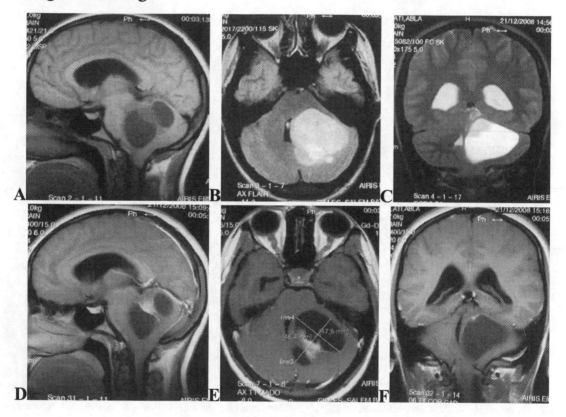

MR Scan pre-contrast sagittal T1 (A), axial FLAIR (B), coronal T2 (C), post-contrast sagittal (D), axial (E) and coronal (F) T1-weighted images reveal a large biloculated left cerebellar cystic mass of low-T1 and high-FLAIR and T2 signal intensity, containing a small solid enhanced nodule with mild peripheral vasogenic edema. The brainstem is compressed and displaced anteriorly with effacement of the pre-pontic cistern; the 4th ventricle is partially obliterated and displaced to the right with tonsilar herniation through the foramen magnum. There is a tri-ventricular obstructive hydrocephalus.

Diagnosis: Pilocytic Astrocytoma

Case 57

Clinical Presentation

A 26 year-old female patient, presented with history of persistent headaches and vomiting.

Radiological Findings

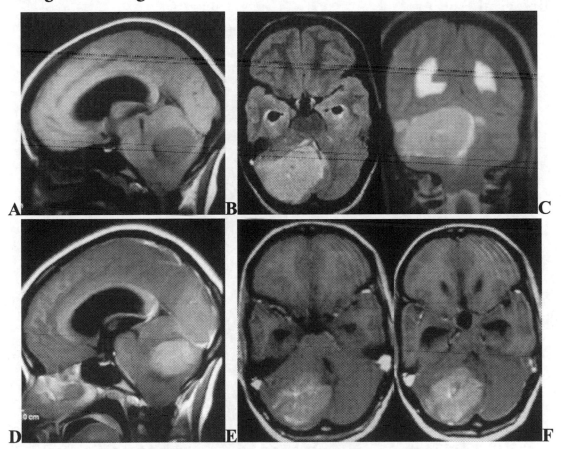

MR Scan, sagittal T1 (A), axial FLAIR (B), coronal T2 (C) and post-contrast sagittal (D) and axial (E, F) T1-weighted images reveal a large intraparenchymal right cerebellar mass of low-T1 and high-FLAIR and T2 signal intensity with intense enhancement after contrast administration, surrounded by small area of vasogenic edema. There is mass effect on the brainstem and 4th ventricle with dilatation of the temporal horns, 3rd and lateral ventricles with mild peri-ventricular interstitial edema.

Diagnosis: Cerebellar Astrocytoma with Obstructive Tri-ventricular Hydrocephalus

Case 58

Clinical Presentation

A 24 year-old female patient with history of headaches and repeated vomiting of three weeks duration.

Radiological Findings

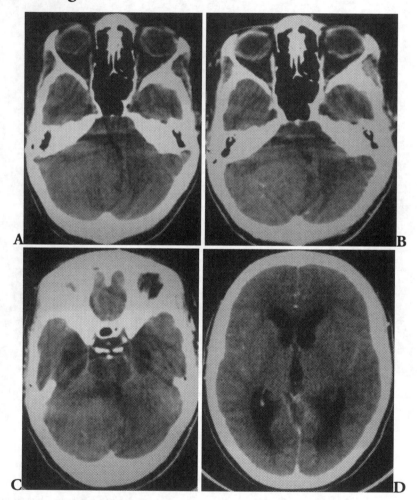

Pre(A)-and post-contrast (B, C, D) brain CT Scan images show a large, oval, well-defined, slightly hyperdense right cerebellar mass with moderate and homogeneous enhancement after contrast administration, compressing and displacing the 4th ventricle and brainstem, obliterating the basal cisterns. Note dilated 3rd and lateral ventricles with periventricular interstitial edema and sulcal effacement.

Diagnosis: Cerebellar Astrocytoma

Case 59

Clinical Presentation

A 4 and ½ year-old male child, presenting abnormal movements.

Radiological Findings

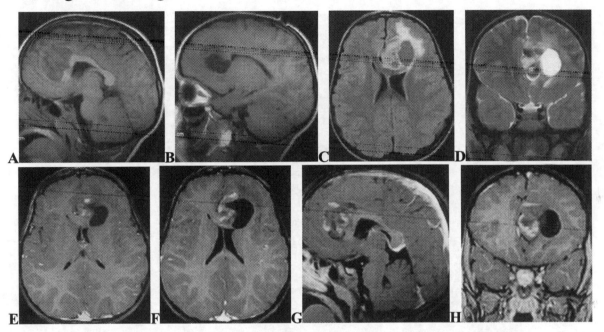

MR Scan, pre-contrast sagittal T1 (A, B), axial FLAIR (C), coronal T2 (D), post-contrast axial (E, F), sagittal (G) and coronal (H) T1-weighted images reveal a left frontal para-sagittal mass with two components, one cystic hypointense on T1, isointense on FLAIR and hyperintense on T2 with no peripheral enhancement and second component is solid slightly hypointense on T1, heterogeneously hyperintense on FLAIR and T2 with heterogeneous enhancement after contrast enhancement. There is mass effect on the corpus callosum, frontal horns and anterior portions of the lateral ventricles.

Diagnosis: Fontal Pilocytic Astrocytoma

Case 60

Clinical Presentation

A 37 year-old female patient with history of chronique headaches.

Radiological Findings

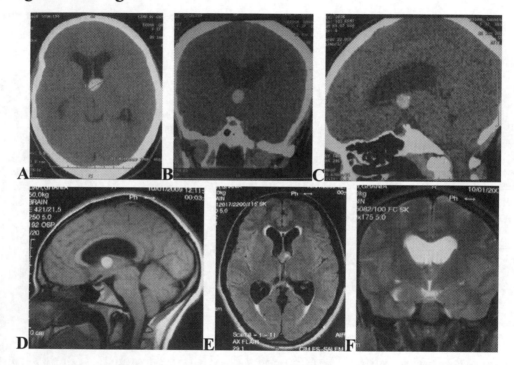

Nonenhanced brain CT Scan axial (A) with coronal (B) and sagittal (C) reconstruction and MR Scan nonenhanced sagittal-T1 (D), axial FLAIR (E) and coronal-T2 (F) images showing a small rounded well defined spontaneously hyperdense lesion of the anterior superior 3rd ventricle obstructing the foramina of Monro with dilated laterale ventricles. On MR, the lesion appears hyperintense on T1 and isointense on FLAIR and T2-weighted images. The lateral ventricles are dilated with mild interstitial peri-ventricular edema seen as high signal on Flair and T2 images.

Diagnosis: Colloid Cyst of 3rd Ventricle with Obstructive Bi-ventricular Hydrocephalus

Case 61

Clinical Presentation

A 12 year-old male with history of repeated vomiting and headaches.

Radiological Findings

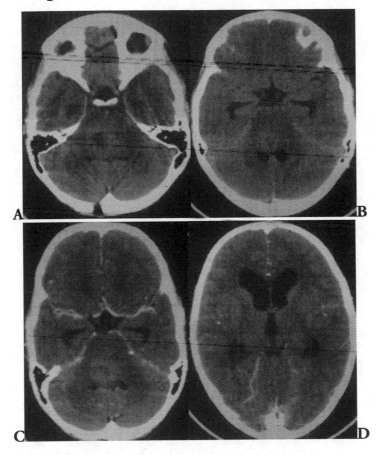

Pre(A, B)-and post-contrast (C, D) brain CT Scan images show a diffusely enlarged hypodense brainstem with focal slightly hyperdense lesion containing central hypodense necrotic area, with mild peripheral enhancement after contrast administration, compressing and displacing the 4th ventricle posteriorly with effacement of the basal cisterns. Note dilated 3rd and lateral ventricles indicating obstructive tri-ventricular hydrocephalus.

Diagnosis: Brainstem glioma

Case 62

Clinical Presentation

A 9 year-old male patient presented with a hemisensory deficit, headaches, nausea and vomiting.

Radiological Findings

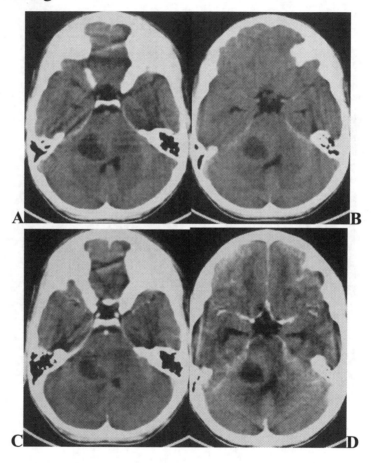

Pre-(A, B) and post-contrast (C, D) brain CT Scan showing an enlarged diffusely hypodense brainstem with an oval cystic mass of its right posterior aspect with ring-like enhancement, compressing and displacing the 4th ventricle with effacement of the posterior fossa cisterns. Note dilated temporal horns indicating raised intra-ventricular pressure..

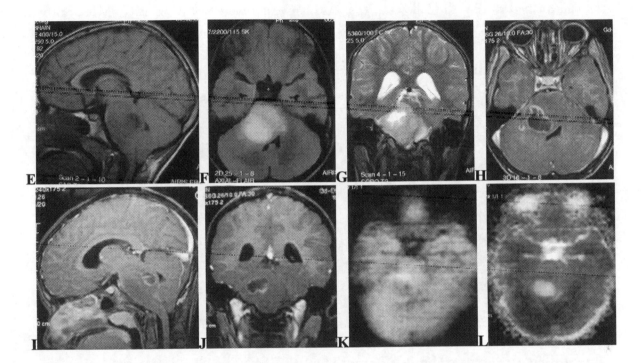

...Continued, MR Scan pre-contrast sagittal T1 (E), axial FLAIR (F), coronal T2 (G), post-contrast axial (H), sagittal (I) and coronal (J) T1-weighted images with DWI-EPI (K) and ADC (L) demonstrate the brainstem lesion as a low-T1 and high-FLAIR and T2 signal intensity lesion with peripheral ring enhancement, surrounded by a large area of brainstem edema with mass effect on the 4th ventricle and tonsilar herniation through the foramen magnum. Note No restricted diffusion (low-signal) with high ADC.

Diagnosis: Brainstem Glioma

Case 63

Clinical Presentation

A 31 year-old male patient, operated for cystic astrocytoma of the posterior fossa. Three CT Scan performed during the follow-up (period of 3 years) were not conclusive. MR Scan was performed to rule out recurrence.

Radiological Findings

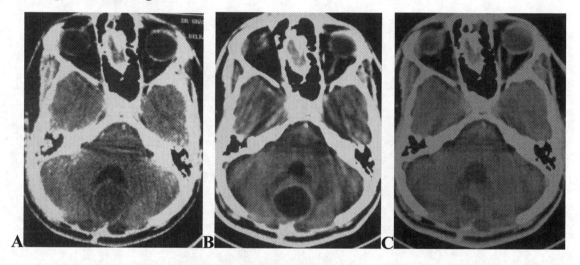

Three differents enhanced brain CT Scan: The 1ˢᵗ CT "A" (done 1 and ½ year after surgery), reveals a small cystic vermian lesion with thin ring enhancement adjacent to the craniotomy and no mass effect on the 4ᵗʰ ventricle. **The 2ⁿᵈ CT Scan "B"** (done 2 and ½ year after surgery) shows that the lesion has approximately the same size and enhancement (stable). **The 3ʳᵈ CT Scan "C"** (done 3 years after surgery) shows that the lesion has significantly decreased in size with still ring enhancement and dilated adjacent 4ᵗʰ ventricle as compared with the 2ⁿᵈ CT Scan.

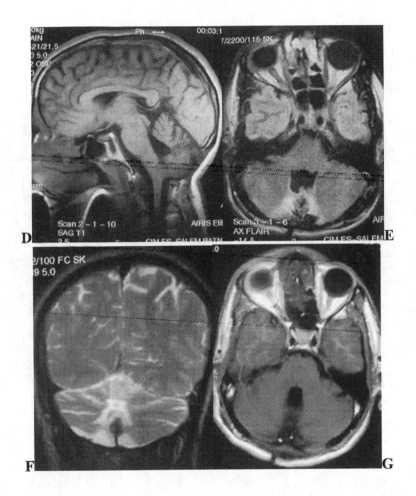

...Continued, MR Scan (done 6 years after surgery), **pre-contrast sagittal T1 (D), axial FLAIR (E), coronal T2 (F) and post-contrast axial T1 (G) images** show a small vermian hypointense area significantly decreased in size as compared with the lateast CT Scan, with no enhancement after gadolinium administration, surrouned by a hyperintense area of gliose and dilated adjacent 4th ventricle, indicating a Postoperative Cavity with no recurrence.

Diagnosis: Postoperative Cavity

Case 64

Clinical Presentation

A 52 year-old male patient, with history of bilateral papilledema and left hemiparesis.

Radiological Findings

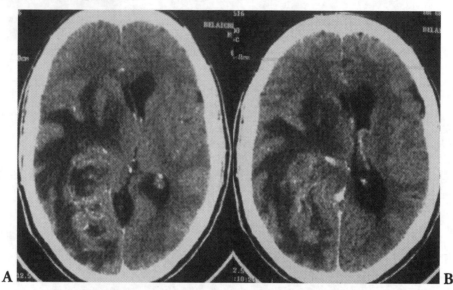

Enhanced brain CT Scan demonstrates a large, lobulated, intraparenchymal tumoral mass of the right temporo-parietal region, heterogeneously enhanced after contrast administration with central hypodense necrotic area, surrounded by large area of vasogenic edema, obliterating the adjacent lateral ventricle with midline shift to the left.

Diagnosis: Glioblastoma

Case 65

Clinical Presentation

A 62 year-old male patient with history of recent seizures.

Radiological Findings

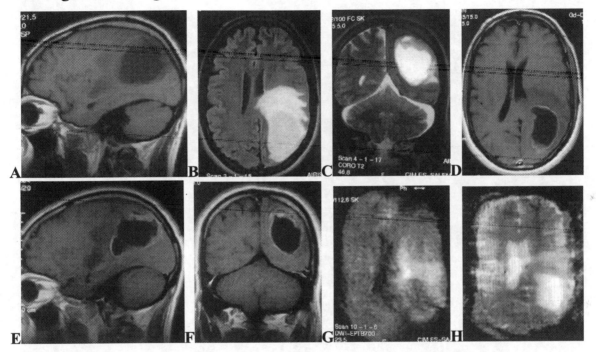

MR Scan, pre-contrast sagittal T1 (A), axial FLAIR (B), coronal T2 (C), post-contrast axial (D), sagittal (E), and coronal (F)-T1, and DWI-EPI-PG (G) with ADC (H) showing a large intra-axial mass of the left occipito-parietal region of low-T1 and high FLAIR and T2 signal intensity with thick and irregular ring enhancement. The DWI image shows no restriction within the lesion (hyposignal) with high ADC. There is a significant vasogenic edema around the lesion with sulcal effacement and obliteration of the adjacent portion of the lateral ventricle.

Diagnosis: Glioblastoma

Case 66

Clinical Presentation

A 56 year-old male patient with frontal syndrome.

Radiological Findings

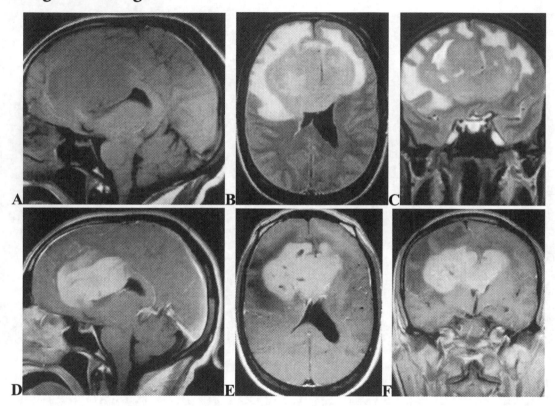

MR Scan pre-contrast sagittal T1 (A), axial FLAIR (B), coronal T2 (C), post-contrast sagittal (D), axial (E) and coronal (F)) T1-weighted images reveal a large bilateral fronto-callosal tumoral process, with irregular lobulated contours, involving the anterior interhemispheric fissure and appears of low-T1 and slightly high-T2 and FLAIR signal intensity, containing central areas of necrosis or cystic degeneration. After gadolinium administration the lesion shows intense enhancement of its solid component. Note a large surrounding area of vasogenic edema with mass effect on the frontal horns and anterior portion of the lateral ventricles.

Diagnosis: Fronto-Callosal Glioblastoma

Case 67

Clinical Presentation

A 69 year-old hypertensive male patient, presented with right hemiparesis.

Radiological Findings

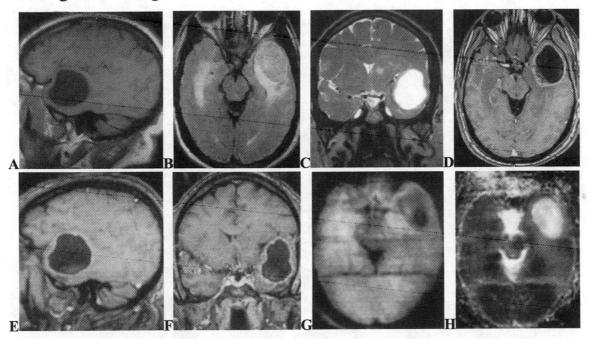

MR Scan pre-contrast sagittal T1 (A), axial FLAIR (B), coronal T2 (C) and post-contrast axial (D), sagittal (E) and coronal (F) T1-weighted images with DWI-EPI-PG (G) and ADC (H) showing an oval intra-axial left temporal lesion, which appears hypointense on T1, isointense on FLAIR and hyperintense on T2 with irregular ring enhancement after gadolinium administration, surrounded by mild area of vasogenic edema, obliterating the adjacent temporal horn. On diffusion image the lesion shows low signal (no restriction) with high ADC.

Diagnosis: Cystic Glioblastoma

Case 68

Clinical Presentation

A 35 year-old with progressive personality changes and mental status disturbance.

Radiological Findings

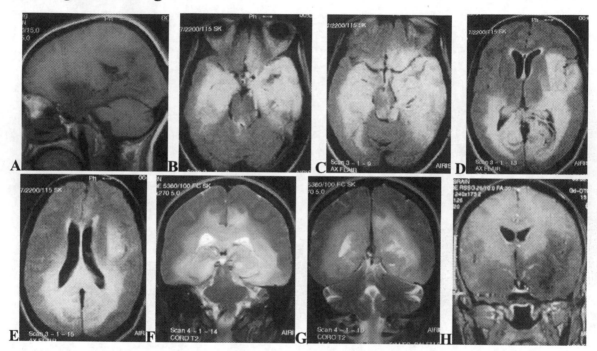

MR Scan pre-contrast sagittal T1 (A), axial FLAIR (B, C, D, E), coronal T2 (F, G), and post-contrast coronal (H)) T1-weighted images: Extensive low-T1 and high-FLAIR and T2 signal intensity with mass effect is noted throughout the temporal and occipital lobes, left frontal lobe and insular region (involving white and gray matter), splenium of corpus callosum and peri-ventricular white matter and partially the brainstem, with no enhancement after gadolinium administration.

Diagnosis: Gliomatosis Cerebri

Case 69

Clinical Presentation

A 22 year-old male patient with 3 years history of temporal epilepsy.

Radiological Findings

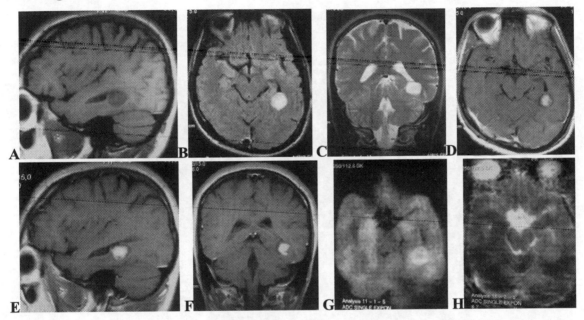

Scan pre-contrast sagittal T1 (A), axial FLAIR (B), coronal T2 (C), post-contrast axial (D), sagittal (E) and coronal (F) T1-weighted images with DWI-EPI (G) and ADC (H): there is a small rounded well-defined low-T1 and high-FLAIR and T2 lesion of the left temporal lobe of postero-inferior location, with intense and homogeneous enhancement after gadolinium administration, surrounded by thin rim of vasogenic edema. Note mild mass effect on the adjacent temporal horn. On diffusion image the lesion shows high signal (restricted diffusion) with high ADC.

Diagnosis: Ganglioglioma

Case 70

Clinical Presentation

A 21 year-old male patient presented with history of epilepsy.

Radiological Findings

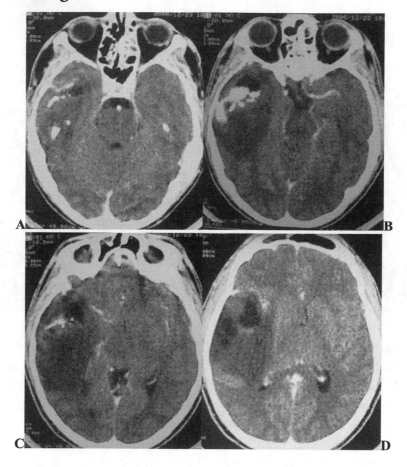

Enhanced brain CT Scan showing a large right intra-axial hypodense temporo-frontal tumoral process containing cystic area and calcifications, with no significant enhancement. There is a complete obliteration of the right temporal horn and partially of the lateral ventricle and basal citerns with mild shifted midline structures.

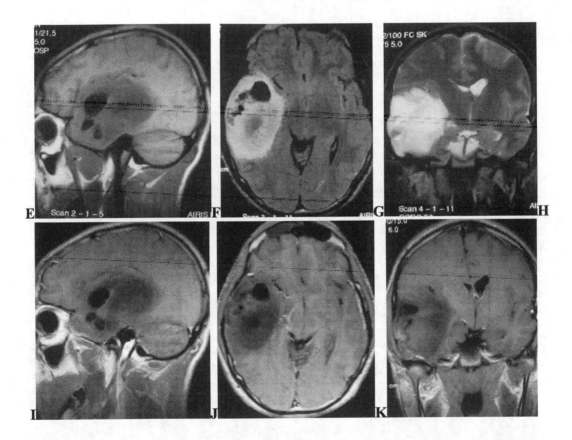

...continued, **MR Scan, pre-contrast sagittal T1 (E), axial FLAIR (F), coronal T2 (G), post-contrast sagittal (I), axial (J) and coronal (K) T1-weighted images:** The right temporo-frontal lesion appears hypointense on T1, hyperintense on FLAIR and T2 with a small cystic component of low-T1 and FLAIR and high T2 and foci of calcifications hypointense on all sequences. No significant enhancement of the lesion after gadolinium administration.

Diagnosis: Oligodendroglioma (Grade A)

Case 71

Clinical Presentation

A 32 year-old female patient with history of generalized epilepsy.

Radiological Findings

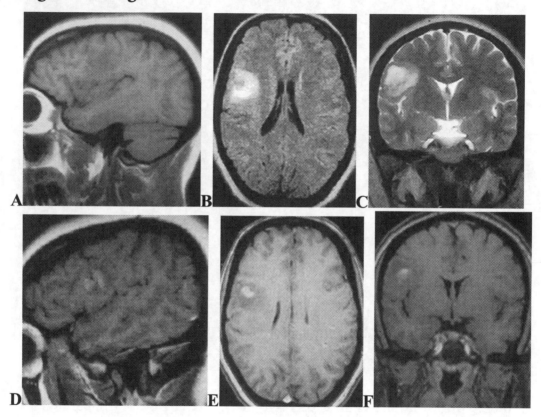

MR Scan pre-contrast sagittal T1 (A), axial FLAIR (B), coronal T2 (C) and post-contrast sagittal (D), axial (E) and coronal (F) T1-weighted images demonstrate a small right frontal lesion, hypointense to the cortical gray matter on T1, isointense on FLAIR and hyperintense on T2 with central nodular enhancement after gadolinium administration, surrounded by area of vasogenic edema hypointense on T1 and hyperintense on FLAIR and T2 images. No significant mass effect on the adjacent sylvian fissure or right lateral ventricle.

Diagnosis: Oligodendroglioma (Grade B)

Case 72

Clinical Presentation

A 54 year-old male patient known case of thoracic Hodgkin's lymphoma., presenting a seizure disorder.

Radiological Findings

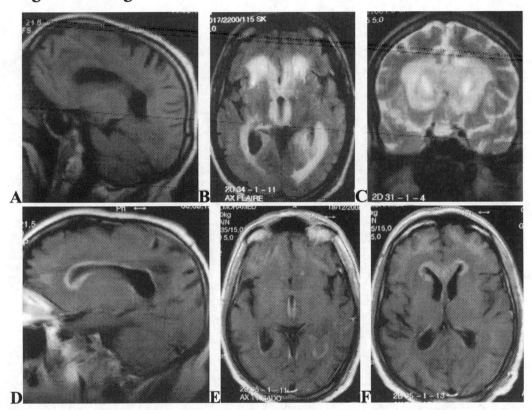

MR Scan , pre-contrast sagittal T1 (A), axial FLAIR (B), coronal T2 (C), post-contrast sagittal and axial (D, E, F) T1-weighted images showing a thickened wall of the ventricular system which appears of low-T1 and high-T2 and FLAIR with intense enhancement after gadolinium administration, surrounded by an area peri-ventricular white matter edema. Note involvement of the corpus callosum.

Diagnosis: Secondary Cerebral Lymphoma

Case 73

Clinical Presentation

A 57 year-old male patient,, known case of nasopharyngeal Ca. treated since two years by radiotherapy, presented with right visual field anomalies.

Radiological Findings

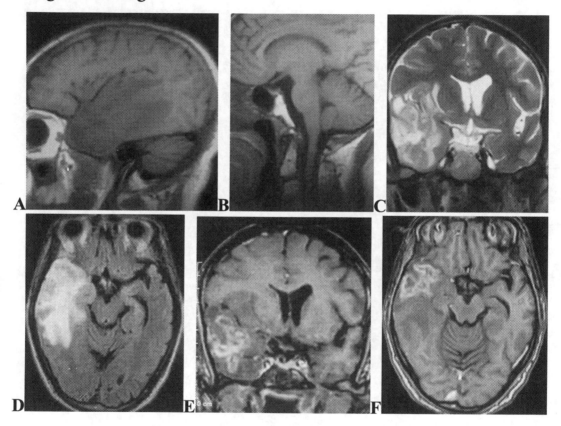

MR Scan, pre-contrast sagittal T1 (A, B), coronal T2 (C), axial FLAIR (D), and post-contrast coronal (E) and axial (F) T1-weighted images showing a large low-T1 and high-FLAIR and T2 lesion with heterogeneous enhancement after gadolinium administration located in the right temporal lobe, and surrounded by area of edema with mass effect on the ipsilateral temporal horn. Note the hyperintense appearance of the clivus C1 and C2 (fatty degeneration usually seen after radiotherapy).

Diagnosis: Cerebral Radionecrosis with Fatty Degeneration of the Clivus, C1 and C2

Case 74

Clinical Presentation

A 63 year-old female patient with spastic tetraparesis.

Radiological Findings

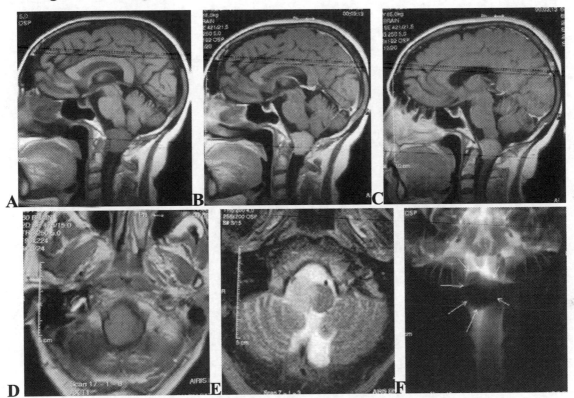

MR Scan Pre-contrast sagittal (A)-and postcontrast sagittal (B, C), and axial (D) T1 and T2 (E)-weighted images with myelo-MR (F) showing an intra-dural extra-medullary lesion filling the right side of the foramen magnum at the level of the bulbo-medullary junction. This lesion appears of low-T1, high-T2 with strong and homogeneous enhancement after contrast administration and as a filling defect on the myelo-MR, compressing and displacing the bulbo-medullary junction to the left.

Diagnosis: Meningioma at Foramen Magnum

Case 75

Clinical Presentation

A 55 year-old female patient with right sided hearing deficit. On physical exam. decreased hearing on right.

Radiological Findings

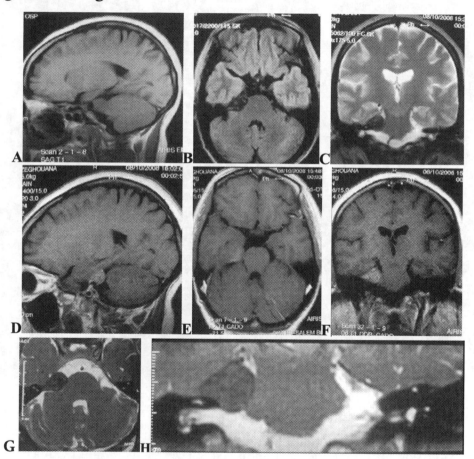

MR Scan pre-contrast sagittal T1 (A), axial FLAIR (B), coronal T2 (C), post-contrast sagittal (D), axial (E) and coronal (F) and axial /coronal GE-BASG (G, H): there is a broad based extra-axial mass located in the right cerebello-pontine angle, antero-superior to the acoustic-facial complex, extending to the porous acousticus but not entering the internal auditory canal. The mass demonstrates isointensity relative to gray matter on T1-weighted and decreased signal on FLAIR and T2-weighted sequences. The mass enhances homogeneously with contrast and presenting a dural tail centered on posterior petrous wall.

Diagnosis: CPA Meningioma

Case 76

Clinical Presentation

A 67 year-old male patient admitted to the psychiatric ward by family members. Her complaints included weakness, depressed mood, and new-onset urinary incontinence

Radiological Findings

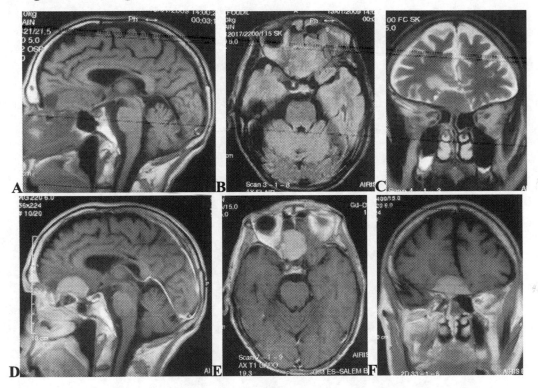

Brain MR Scan pre-contrast sagittal (A), axial FLAIR (B), coronal T2 (C) and post-contrast sagittal (D), axial (E), and coronal (F) images reveal a midline extra-axial mass at the base of frontal region, arising from the cribriform palate. This mass appears isointense to the white matter on T1 and T2-weighted images and slightly hyperintense on FLAIR with localized area of edema seen anteriorly. After contrast administration the lesion shows an intense and homogeneous enhancement. Note that on T2 coronal image the lesion is surrounded by a thin hyperintense rim of CSF indicating its extra-axial location in addition to its broad-base.

Diagnosis: Olfactory Groove Meningioma

Case 77

Clinical Presentation

This 68 year-old man presented with a history of a subtle change in personality, less spontaneous activity, and mild difficulty with memory.

Radiological Findings

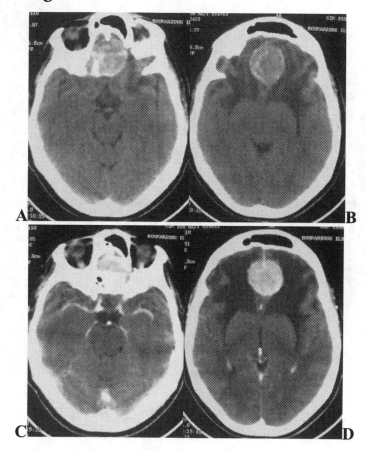

Pre-(A, B) and post-contrast (C, D) brain CT Scan, shows an oval extra-axial, slightly hyperdense mass, containing areas of calcification, located in the midline floor of the anterior cranial fossa, with intense and homogeneous enhancement after contrast administration. There is a vasogenic edema around the lesion, in both frontal lobes, obliterating the frontal horns.

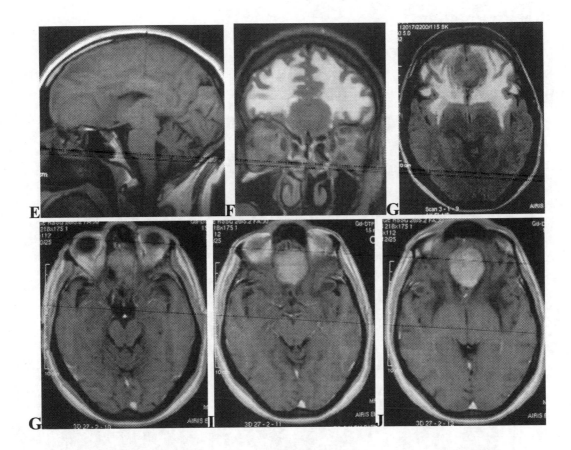

…continued, MR Scan, pre-contrast sagittal (E), coronal T2 (F), axial FLAIR (G) and post-contrast axial (G, I, J) images confirm the presence of a midline extra-axial mass at the base of frontal region, arising from the cribriform palate, which appears isointense to the gray matter on T1, T2 and FLAIR images with large area of vasogenic edema around the lesion, obliterating the frontal horns. After contrast administration the lesion shows an intense and homogeneous enhancement. Note that on sagittal T1 the frontal lobe is displaced superiorly and posteriorly and on T2 coronal image the lesion is surrounded by a thin hyperintense rim of CSF indicating its extra-axial location in addition to its broad-base.

Diagnosis: Olfactory Groove Meningioma

Case 78

Clinical Presentation

A 62 year-old female patient with left hemiparesis.

Radiological Findings

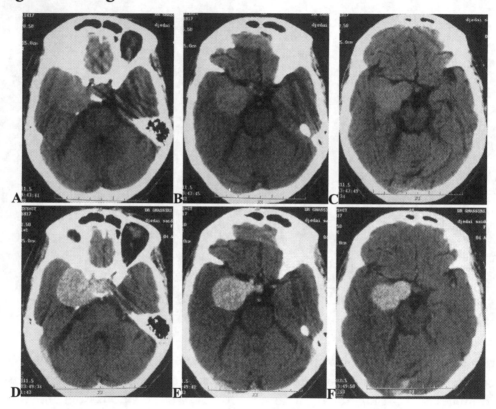

Pre-(A, B, C) and post-contrast (D, E, F) brain CT Scan showing a large rounded well-defined spontaneously hyperdense extra-axial mass of the right cavernous sinus with intense and homogeneous enhancement after contrast administration, encircling partially the right intracavernous ICA with extension to the sellar region and right side of the opto-chiasmatic cisten. Note also extension to the homolateral temporal fossa obliterating the temporal horn. On bone settings (not shown) there is erosion of the right orbital apex and right anterior clinoid process.

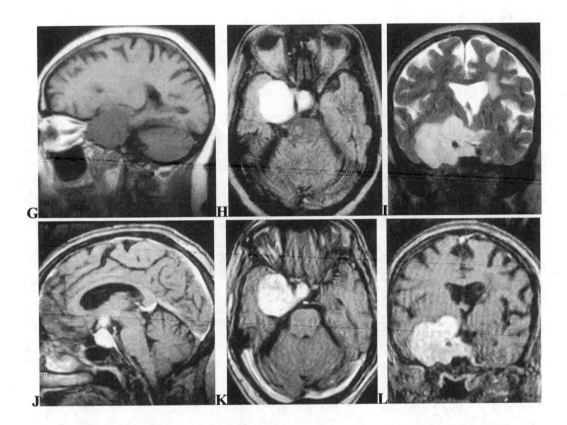

...continued, MR Scan pre-contrast sagittal T1 (G), axial FLAIR (H), coronal T2 (I), post-contrast sagittal (J), axial (K) and coronal (L)) T1-weighted images: The right cavernous sinus mass appears of low-T1, high-FLAIR and T2 signal intensity with strong and homogeneous enhancement after gadolinium administration, surrounding the intracavernous ICA which shows reduced caliber as compared to the left side with superior displacement. Note extension of the lesion to sellar and right supra-sellar regions, filling partially the opto-chiasmatic cistern.

Diagnosis: Cavernous Sinus Meningioma

Case 79

Clinical Presentation

An 82 year-old female patient with history of chronic headache.

Radiological Findings

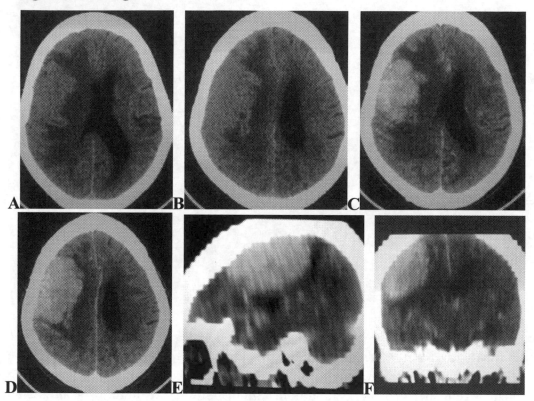

Pre-(A, B)-and post-contrast (C, D) CT Scan with sagittal (E) and coronal (F) reconstruction showing a large right frontal pre-central extra-axial mass, isodense to the cortical gray matter with intense and homogeneous enhancement. The extra-axial location is evidenced by the broad-based attachment to the adjacent dura. There is perilesional vasogenic edema obliterating the adjacent lateral ventricle with dilated contralateral lateral ventricle.

Diagnosis: Frontal Meningioma

Case 80

Clinical Presentation

A 37 year-old female patient with 18 months history of epilepsy. The clinical examination reveals a right hemiparesis.

Radiological Findings

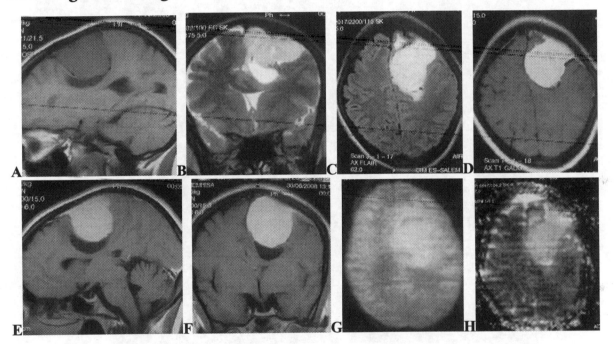

MR Scan, pre-contrast sagittal T1 (A), coronal T2 (B), axial FLAIR (C), post-contrast axial (D), sagittal (E) and coronal (F) weighted images with DWI-EPI (G) and ADC (H) images show a large left para-sagittal extra-axial mass with broad-based attachment to the dura of the adjacent frontal convexity. This mass shows low-T1 and high-FLAIR and T2 signal intensity with intense and homogeneous enhancement after gadolinium administration with thin rim of CSF between the lesion and cerebral parenchyma, indicating its extra-axial location. There is a cystic component inferior to the lesion of low-T1 and high T2 signal intensity and mass effect on the body of the corpus callosum and left LV. On DWI image the lesion shows restricted diffusion with high ADC.

Diagnosis: Meningioma of the Frontal Convexity with Cystic Component

Case 81

Clinical Presentation

A 46 year-old female patient with history of frontal lobe syndrome.

Radiological Findings

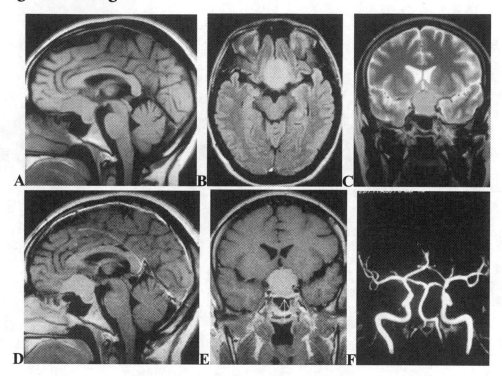

MR Scan, pre-contrast sagittal (A), axial FLAIR (B), coronal T2 (C), post-contrast sagittal and coronal (D, E) and MRA-3D-TOF (F): showing a well-defined extra-axial mass of the anterior skull base in contact the jugum of the sphenoid and optic gutter with posterior extension, filling the sellar and supra-sellar region. This mass appears isointense to the cortical gray matter on T1 and T2 and hyperintense on FLAIR sequence with intense and homogeneous enhancement after gadolinium administration. The pituitary gland is well-visualized (white arrow), compressed against the sellar floor, excluding the possibility of macroadenoma. The pituitary stalk and optic chiasma are displaced posteriorly. On coronal images (C, E) and on MRA there is definite regular narrowing the left supra-clinoid portion of the ICA and A1 segment of the ACA.

Diagnosis: Meningioma of the Jugum and Optic Gutter

Case 82

Clinical Presentation

A 50 year-old female patient presented with two years history of headaches, gait disturbance and one month history of vomitting and dizziness. Neurological examination revealed bilateral papilledema, dysmetria and ataxia.

Radiological Findings

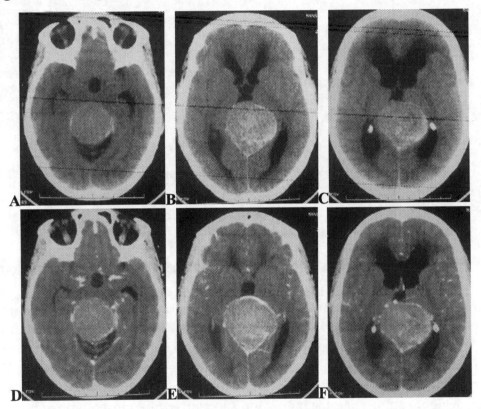

Pre-contrast (A, B, C) and post-contrast (D, E, F) CT Scan demonstrates a large rounded well-defined spontaneously hyperdense mass of the pineal region with intense and homogeneous enhancement after contrast administration in contact with the tentorium cerebella, which appears thickened and enhanced mainly the left edge. There is marked compression of the brainstem and posterior portion of the 3rd ventricle with secondary tri-ventricular obstructive hydrocephalus and interstitial peri-ventricular edema.

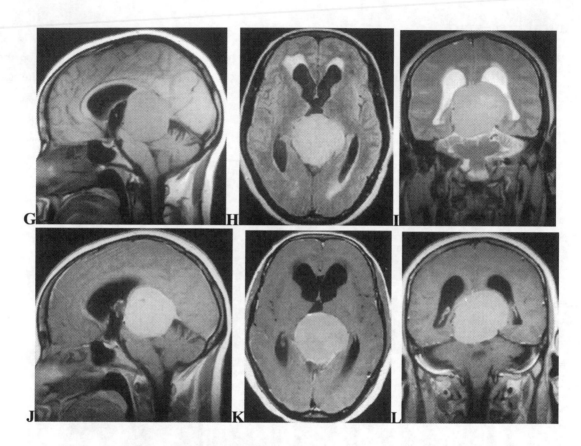

...continued, MR Scan pre-contrast sagittal T1 (G), axial FLAIR (H), coronal T2 (I) and post-contrast sagittal (J), axial (K) and coronal (L) T1-weighted images showing the previously described mass of the pineal region, which appears isointense on T1, hyperintense on FLAIR and T2 sequences with strong and homogeneous enhancement after gadolinium administration. This mass appears in contact with the tentorium cerebelli and extending to the pineal region, compressing the brainstem, superior vermis and posterior portion of the 3rd ventricle which appears displaced anteriorly. As seen on CT Scan there is a secondary obstructive tri-ventricular hydrocephalus with interstitial peri-ventricular edema.

Diagnosis: Meningioma of Pineal Region

Case 83

Clinical Presentation

A 64 year-old female patient with history of chronic headaches and recent episodes of convulsions. Clinical examination shows features of raised intracranial pressure,.

Radiological Findings

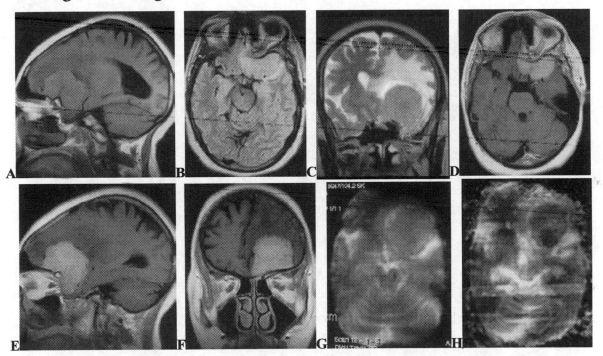

MR Scan pre-contrast sagittal (A), axial FLAIR (B), coronal T2 (C) and post-contrast axial (D), sagittal (E), and coronal (F) with DWI-EPI (G) and ADC (H) showing a left temporo-frontal extra-axial mass centered on the left sphenoid wing with a large broad-based dural attachment. This mass appears isointense to the white matter on T1 and T2 images, slightly hyperintense on FLAIR and DWI with low ADC and shows intense and homogeneous enhancement after gadolinium administration, surrounded by area of vasogenic edema. There is mass effect on the left frontal horn and 3rd ventricle with dilated lateral ventricles. On MRA 3D-TOF (not shown), the left ACA is displaced medially and the MCA posteriorly.

Diagnosis: Sphenoid Wing Meningioma

Case 84

Clinical Presentation

A 36 year-old female complaining of headaches with progressive swelling of the median frontoparietal region.

Radiological Findings

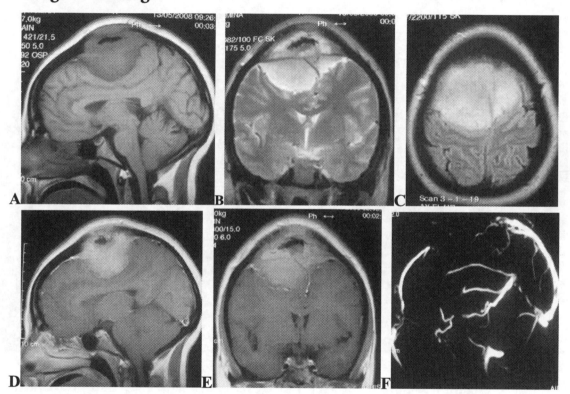

MR Scan, pre-contrast sagittal (A)-T1, coronal (E)-T2, axial FLAIR (C), post-contrast sagittal (D) and coronal (E)-T1 and MRV-2D-TOF(F) images showing a large, median frontoparietal broad-based extra-axial tumoral mass of low-T1 and high-T2-and FLAIR signal intensity with a central hypointense area (calcification), intensely enhanced by contrast administration with evidence of dural thickening (dural-tail).. This tumoral process compresses and displaces the adjacent cerebral parenchyma inferiorly, invades the superior sagittal sinus with destruction of the adjacent cranial vault superiorly.

Diagnosis: Meningioma of Cerebral Convexity

Case 85

Clinical Presentation

A 29 year-old female patient with history a chronic headaches and recent episodes of vomiting.

Radiological Findings

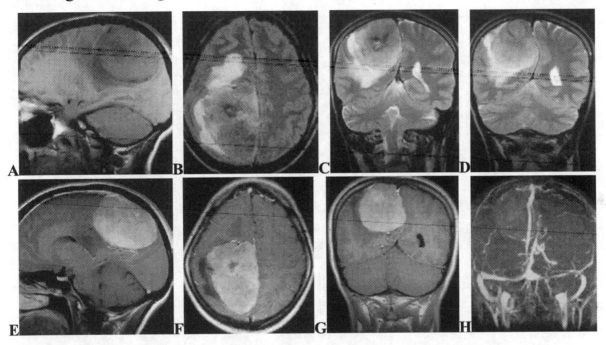

MR Scan pre-contrast sagittal T1 (A), axial FLAIR (B), coronal T2 (C, D), post-contrast sagittal (E), axial (F), coronal (G) T1-weighted images with MRV-2D-TOF (H) reveal a large extra-axial mass of right parietal para-sagittal location with broad-based attachment to the falx cerebri, in contact with the parietal convexity This mass appears isointense to the cortical gray matter on T1, T2 and FLAIR with intense and homogeneous enhancement except the central foci of calcifications which appears hypointense in all sequences. Note the thin hyperintense rim of CSF surrounding the mass well-visualized on coronal T2 images indicating with the broad-based attachment, the extra-axial location of the mass. There is a peripheral vasogenic edema obliterating partially the ipsilatral LV with mass effect on the splenium of corpus callosum and falx cerebri. The MRV doesn't show extension to the superior sagittal sinus.

Diagnosis: Meningioma of Falx Cerebri

Case 86

Clinical Presentation

A 56 year-old female patient presented with left exophthalmia.

Radiological Findings

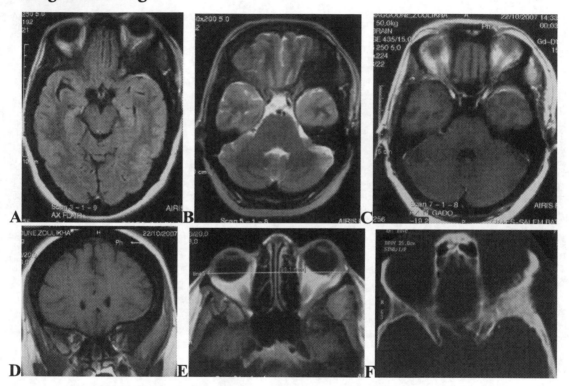

MR Scan axial FLAIR (A), and T2 (B), post-contrast-contrast axial (C, E), coronal (D)-T1, and axial CT Scan bone setting (F), showing a small arciform extra-axial lesion of the left temporal fossa, which appears hyperintense on FLAIR, isointense on T2 with strong enhancement after contrast administration. The adjacent sphenoid wing shows hyperostosis with marked hypointensity (hyperostosis with densification on CT), reducing the left orbital volume with axial exophthalmos grade II.

Diagnosis: Meningioma en Plaque

Case 87

Clinical Presentation

A 63 year-old female patient, presented with right exophthalmia.

Radiological Findings

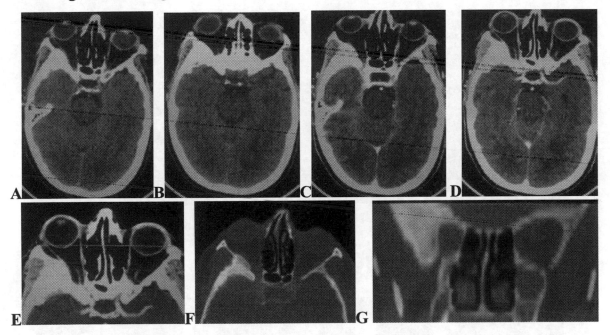

Pre-(A, B) and post-contrast (C, D, E) CT Scan with bone setting and coronal recorstruction (F, G) showing foci of extraparenchymal calcification in the anterior portion of the right temporal fossa. After contrast administration there is evidence of a small arciform extra-axial lesion with strong and homogeneous enhancement. The adjacent sphenoid wing shows a hyperostosis with densification, reducing the right orbital volume with axial exophthalmos grade I.

Diagnosis: Meningioma En Plaque

Case 88

Clinical Presentation

A 44 year-old female patient presented with strabism and left VI nerve palsy.

Radiological Findings

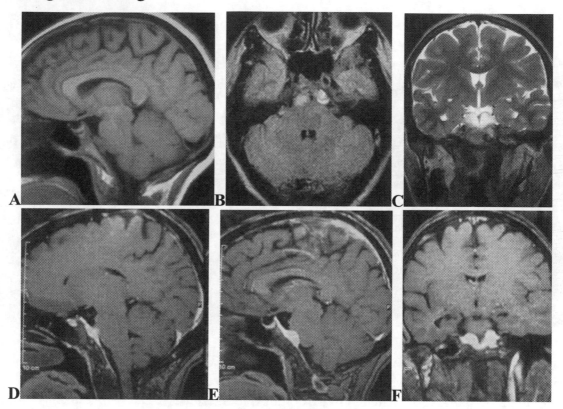

MR Scan pre-contrast sagittal T1 (A), axial FLAIR (B), coronal T2 (C) and post-contrast sagittal (D, E) and coronal (F) T1-weighted images reveal a retro-clival, pre-pontic bilobulated extra-axial mass, developed on both sides of midline with broad-based area in contact with the clivus. This mass appears slightly hypointense on T1, hyperintense on FLAIR and T2 with intense and homogeneous enhancement after gadolinium administration with mild mass effect on the pons. The left 6th nerve were not visible in its cisternal course most likely compressed. Note the broad-based area of the mass in contact with the clivus and dural enhancement.

Diagnosis: Retro-clival Meningioma

Case 89

Clinical Presentation

A 40 year-old male patient with history of chronic headache.

Radiological Findings

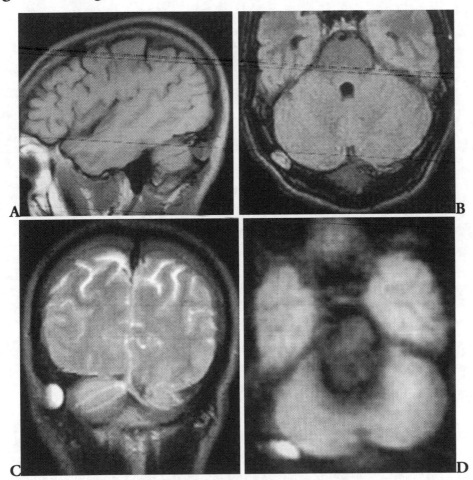

Nonenhanced MR Scan sagittal T1 (A), axial FLAIR(B), coronal T2 (C), and Diffusion (D) weighted images show a small oval well-defined right occipital intradiploic lesion of low-T1, and high-FLAIR, T2 and DWI. No other brain abnormality.

Diagnosis: Intradiploic Epidermoid Cyst

Case 90

Clinical Presentation

A 5 year-old male child with swelling of the mid-upper frontal region;

Radiological Findings

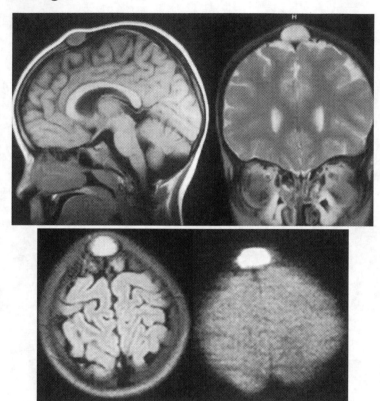

MR Scan sagittal T1 (A), coronal T2 (B), axial FLAIR (C) and DWI-EPI (D) showing a small oval well-defined intradiploic lesion at the mid-frontal region of low-T1 and high-T2, FLAIR and diffusion. There is thinning of the inner and outer table of skull with no obliteration of the adjacent superior sagittal sinus.

Diagnosis: Intradiploic Epidermoid Cyst

Case 91

Clinical Presentation

An 18 year-old female, complaining of chronic headaches.

Radiological Findings

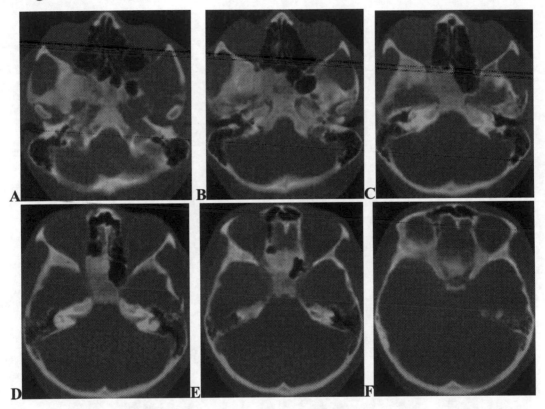

Brain CT Scan (bone settings) shows thickening with osteosclerosis giving a "ground-glass" appearance of the body and horizontal portion of the greater wing of the right sphenoid and the clivus. No cerebral lesion seen on parenchymal window (not shown).

Diagnosis: Right Sphenoid Fibrous Dysplasia

Case 92

Clinical Presentation

A 26 year-old female patient with galactorrhea, irregular periods and hyperprolactinemia.

Radiological Findings

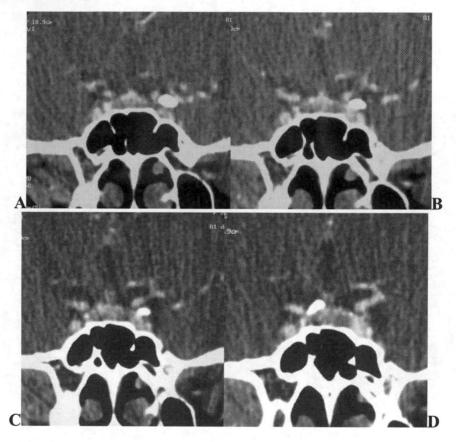

Dynamic Enhanced coronal CT Scan with 2 mm thin cuts of the pituitary gland showing a small (8 mm), rounded, well-defined left parasagittal focal hypodense pituitary lesion, less enhanced than the normal pituitary gland with convex appearance of the upper sellar diaphragm and shifted infundibulum to the right. No sellar floor ersion on bone settings (not shown).

Diagnosis: Pituitary Microadenoma (Prolactinoma)

Case 93

Clinical Presentation

A 29 year-old male patient with high prolactin level.

Radiological Findings

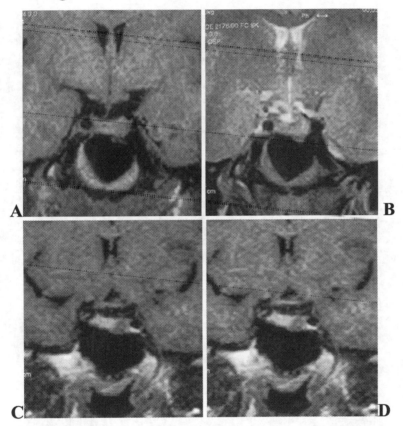

MR Scan, Pre-contrast coronal T1 (A) and T2 (B) and post-contrast dynamic (C, D) T1-weighted images of the sellar region demonstrate a small (9 mm) rounded left para-central lesion of the pituitary gland of low-T1 before and after gadolinium administration and slightly high-T2. The pituitary stalk is slightly shifted to the right. Note mild thinning of the adjacent pituitary floor with no destruction or extension to the sphenoid sinus.

Diagnosis: Microadenoma (Prolactinoma)

Case 94

Clinical Presentation

A 34 year-old female patient with amenorrhea, galactorrhea and hyperprolactinemia.

Radiological Findings

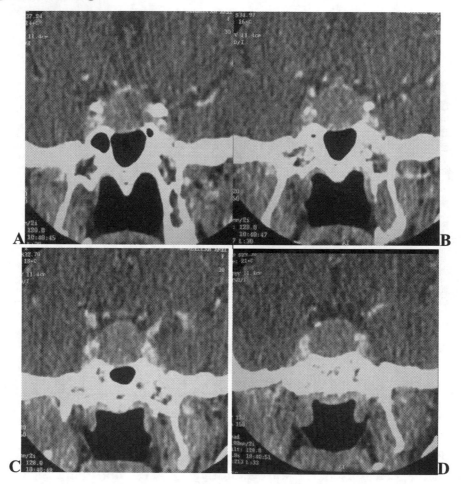

Enhanced CT Scan of the sellar region reveals a rounded well-defined intra-sellar hypodense mass (18 mm of diameter in this case) surrounded by a thin rim of a pituitary tissue with supra-sellar extension, filling the opto-chiasmatic cistern and not compressing the optic chiasma. The pituitary stalk is not visible. Note the destruction of the sellar floor with no infra-sellar nor cavernous sinuses extension.

Diagnosis: Pituitary Macroadenoma (Secreting Prolactinoma)

Case 95

Clinical Presentation

A 48 year-old female patient with history vertigo and hyperprolatinemia.

Radiological Findings

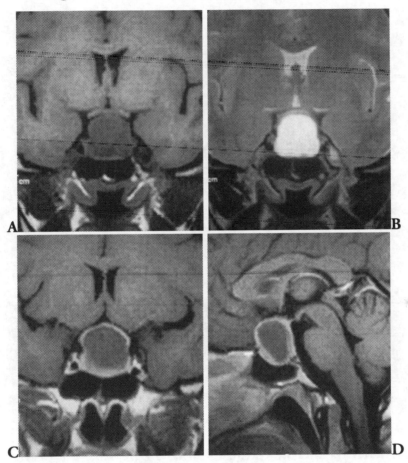

MRI Scan, pre-contrast coronal T1 (A), coronal T2 (B), and post-contrast coronal (C) and sagittal (D) T1- weighted images showed a Large, low-T1 and high-T2 eight-shaped intra-and supra-sellar lesion with homogeneous content, not enhanced after gadolinium administration, surrounded by thin rim of pituitary tissue, filling the opto-chiasmatic cistern, compressing the optic chiasma and pituitary stalk. No infra-sellar extension.

Diagnosis: Macroprolactinoma (fluid content)

Case 96

Clinical Presentation

A 26 year-old female patient with history of severe headaches.

Radiological Findings

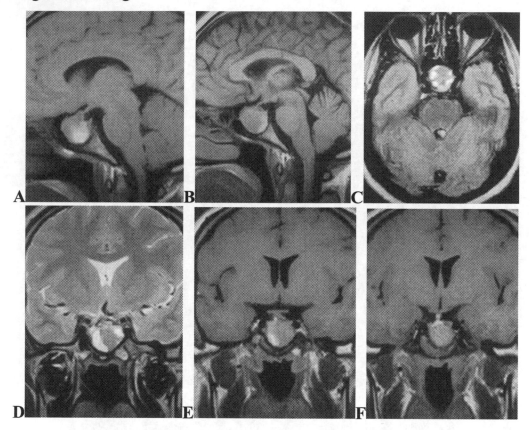

MR Scan of the sellar region, pre-contrast sagittal T1 (A, B), axial FLAIR (C), coronal T2 and post-contrast coronal T1 (E, F) images demonstrate a well-defined intra-sellar soft tissue mass with supra-sellar extension, filling the opto-chiasmatic cistern. This mass shows an isointense signal on T1, T2 and FLAIR with localized posterior area of high signal intensity on all sequences, indicating a necrotic hemorrhage. After contrast administration there is mild enhancement of the non-necrotic area. The pituitary stalk is shifted to the left. No extension to the cavernous sinuses or infra-sellar region.

Diagnosis: Macroadenoma with Necrotic Hemorrhage

Case 97

Clinical Presentation

A 3 year-old female child with history of epilepsy and recent onset of headaches and vomiting.

Radiological Findings

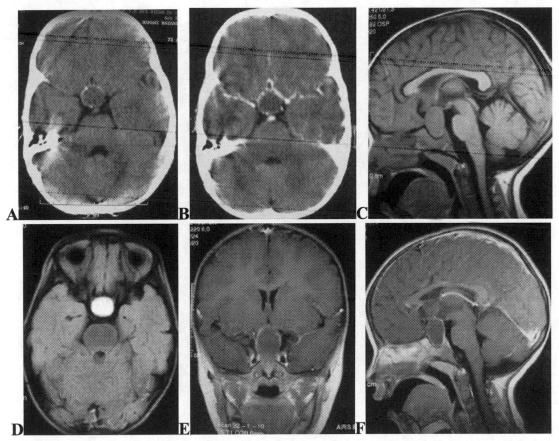

Pre(A)-and postcontrast (B) CT Scan and MR Scan, precontrast sagittal T1 (C), post-contrast coronal and sagittal T1(E, F), and axial FLAIR (D) images: The CT Scan images show a small, rounded well-circumscribed intra-and suprasellar hypodense cystic mass with peripheral rim calcification. On MR sequences the cystic lesion shows oval shape of low-T1 and high-FLAIR with thin and regular rim enhancement. The pituitary gland is flattened against the floor of the sella.

Diagnosis : Craniopharyngioma

Case 98

Clinical Presentation

A 50 year-old female patient with history of vertigo and right hearing loss.

Radiological Findings

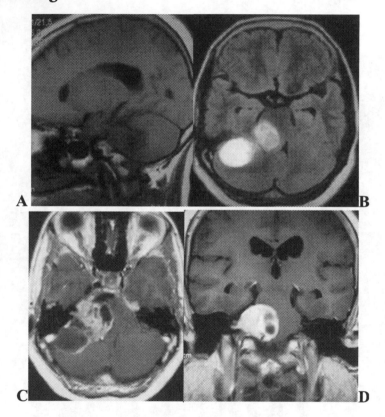

MRI Scan, pre-contrast sagittal T1 (A), axial FLAIR (B), and post-contrast axial (C) & coronal (D)-T1-weighted images showing a large, lobulated, well-defined hypointense T1 and hyperintense FLAIR mass (more than 3 cm), located in the right cerebello-pontine angle, extending into the adjacent internal auditory canal which appears enlarged. There is marked compression and displacement of the brainstem and 4th ventricle to the left side with raised intraventricular pressure. After gadolinium administration the lesion shows strong and homogeneous enhancement with however persistence of hypointense areas (cystic components). Note that the intra-canalar component of the tumor is well-visualized on both axial and coronal images.

Diagnosis: Acoustic Schwannoma Grade IV (Portmann Classification)

Case 99

Clinical Presentation

A 65 year-old male patient presented with right hearing loss and nevralgia in the distribution of the right trigeminal nerve.

Radiological Findings

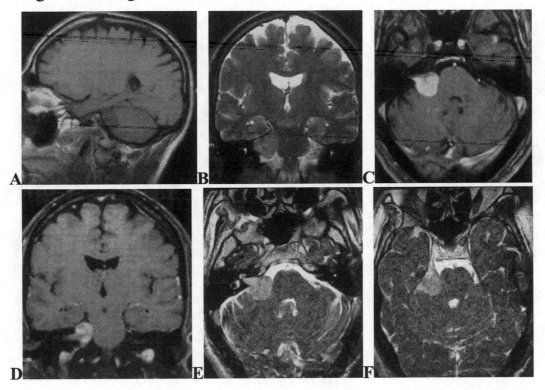

MR Scan pre-contrast sagittal T1 (A), coronal T2 (B) and post-contrast axial (C) and coronal (D) T1-weighted images with axial T*2-BASG (E, F) showing a well-defined low-T1 and slightly high-T2 right cerebello-pontine mass (2.5 cm) with intense enhancement after gadolinium administration, extending into the internal auditory canal, giving the appearance of a scoop of ice-cream on a cone. This mass compresses the brainstem and the emergence of the right trigeminal nerve (as shown on T*2-BASG images) explaining the clinical presentation.

Diagnosis: Acoustic Schwannoma Grade III (Portmann Classification)

Case 100

Clinical Presentation

A 41 year-old male patient presenting with hearing loss, pulsatile tinnitus, bleeding and mass filling the external auditory canal.

Radiological Findings

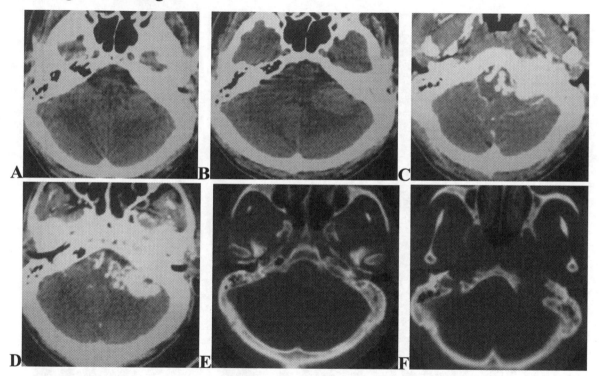

Pre(A, B)-and post-contrast (C, D) brain CT Scan with bone settings (E, F) reveals a large, slightly hyperdense mass, centered on the left jugular foramen with strong and homogeneous enhancement after contrast administration, synchronous to the vascular structures, enlarging the jugular foramen and destructing the jugular process. Anterolaterally the tumor is extended to the left middle ear and EAC, and posteriorly to the cerebello-pontine angle with multiple pre-pontic and surrounding feeding vessels.

Diagnosis: Glomus Jugulotympanicum tumor (Paraganglioma)

Case 101

Clinical Presentation

A 32 year-old male patient presented with right sided pulsatile tinnitus and gradual onset of deafness.

Radiological Findings

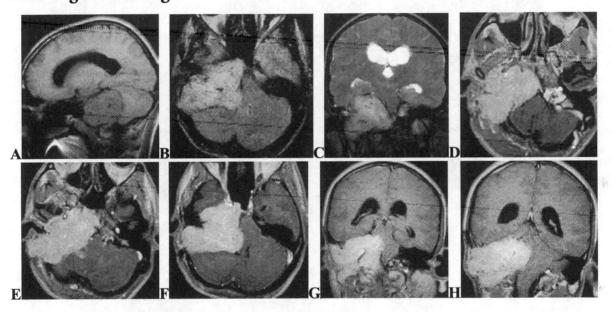

MR Scan pre-contrast sagittal T1 (A), axial FLAIR (B), coronal T2 (C) and post-contrast axial (D, E, F) and coronal (G, H) T1-weighted images showing a huge lobulated jugulo-tympanic extra-axial mass, centered on the jugular foramen and appears slightly hypointense on T1 and hyperintense on FLAIR and T2, containing signal void vascular structures with intense and homogeneous enhancement after gadolinium administration. This lesion shows extension: medially to the cerebello-pontine angle deforming the brainstem and 4th ventricle with tri-ventricular hydrocephalus, antero-superiorly to the middle temporal fossa, displacing the temporal lobe and parapharyngeal space and inferiorly to the carotid and posterior cervical spaces surrounding the jugulo-carotid vascular axis.

Diagnosis: Jugulo-tympanic Paraganglioma

Case 102

Clinical Presentation

A 22 year-old with history severe headaches.

Radiological Findings

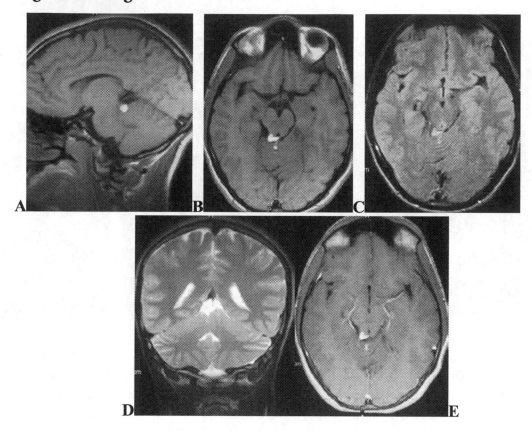

Brain MR, non-enhanced sagittal (A) and axial (B) T1, axial FLAIR (C), coronal T2 (D) and post-contrast axial (E) weighted Images showing a small midline mass in the quadrigeminal cistern, appearing hyperintense on T1, approximately isointense on T2 with some FLAIR hyperintensity. No abnormal enhancement after gadolinium administration.

Diagnosis: Dermoid Cyst

Case 103

Clinical Presentation

A 52 year-old female patient with past-history of left hemiplegia, presented with chronic headaches.

Radiological Findings

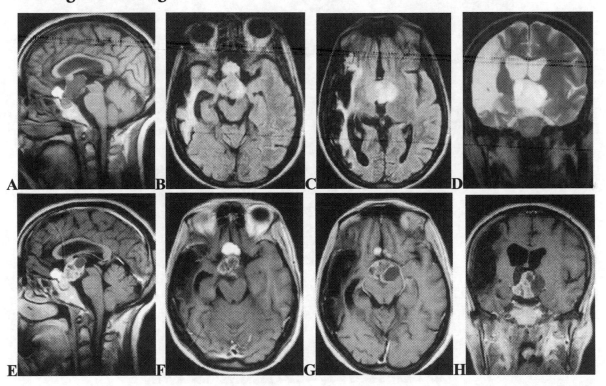

MR Scan, pre-contrast sagittal T1 (A), axial FLAIR (B, C), coronal T2 (D) and post-contrast sagittal (E), axial (F, G) and coronal (H) T1-weighted images reveal a lobulated sellar and supra-sellar mass with three components: a fatty component of anterior location hyperintense on T1, approximately isointense on T2 with some FLAIR hyperintensity; a cystic component with peripheral enhancement and a soft tissue component of sellar and supra-sellar location of low-T1 and high-FLAIR and T2 signal intensity with heterogeneous enhancement after gadolinium administration there is a mass effect on the optic chiasma, and hypothalamus. The pituitary gland is compressed and displaced against the dorsum sellae. Note old infarct in the right middle cerebral artery territory.

Diagnosis: Sellar and Supra-sellar Dermoid Cyst

Case 104

Clinical Presentation

A 47 year-old male patient, known case of nasopharyngeal Carcinoma

Radiological Findings

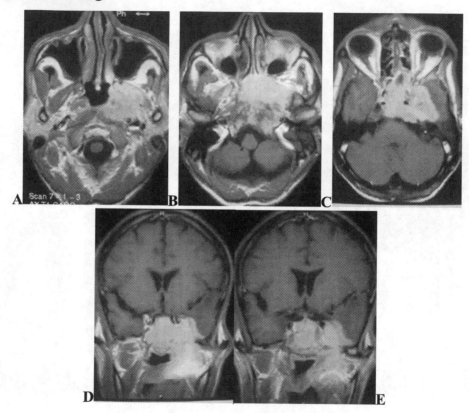

MR Scan, post-contrast axial (A, B, C) and coronal (D, E) T1-weighted images showing a large enhancing tumoral process of the left lateral nasopharyngeal wall. Laterally, obliterating the auditory tube and Rosenmuller fossette, filling the parapharyngeal and pterygoid spaces and infiltrating the pterygoid muscles. Anteriorly, filling partially the posterior part of the ethmoid cells, optic foramina. Posteriorly, partial destruction of the clivus with partial filling of the pre-pontic cistern. Superiorly, note filling of the sphenoid sinus and sellar region with extension of the tumoral process to the internal temporal fossa and left cavernous sinus, encircling the internal carotid artery. Note soft tissue filling the left middle ear and mastoid air cells (oto-mastoiditis).

Diagnosis: Nasopharyngeal Carcinoma (T4)

Malformations, Phacomatosis
and
Granulomatosis

Case 105

Clinical Presentation

A 12 year-old female patient with right facial palsy.

Radiological Findings

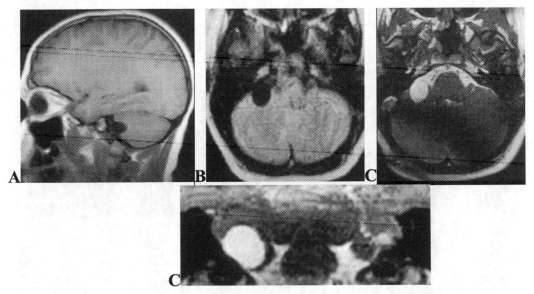

MR Scan, sagittal T1 (A), axial FLAIR (B) and T*2-BASG and coronal T2 (C) showing a small oval extra-axial cystic lesion of identical signal to CSF fluid in all sequences, located in the right cerebello-pontine angle posterior to the acoustic-facial nerves which are displaced anteriorly.

Diagnosis: Arachnoid Cyst of CPA

Case 106

Clinical Presentation

A 42 year-old male patient with history of chronic headaches.

Radiological Findings

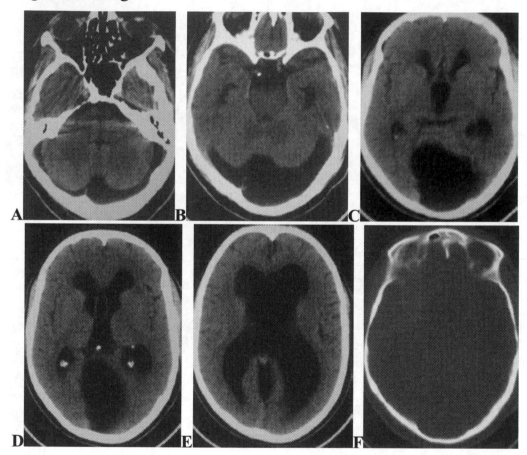

Non-Enhanced brain CT Scan reveals a large retrocerebellar, extra-axial, smoothly marginated cystic mass of CSF density, non-communicating with the 4th ventricle which shows normal size, compressing the brain parenchyma and the aqueduct of Sylvius with triventricular obstructive hydrocephalus Bone settings shows an associated thinning of the inner table of the calvarium.

Diagnosis: Arachnoid Cyst with Obstructive Hydrocephalus

Case 107

Clinical Presentation

A 2 year-old male child with seizures.

Radiological Findings

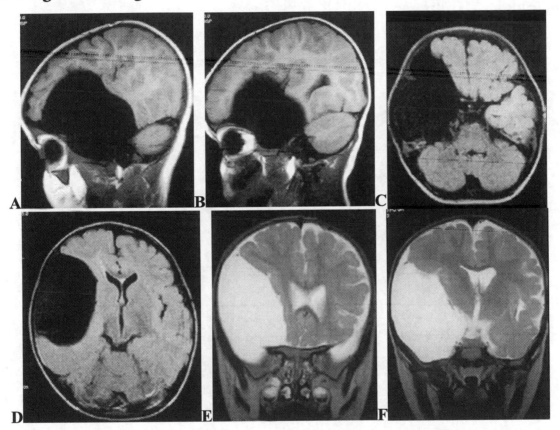

MR Scan sagittal T1 (A , B), axial FLAIR (C, D) and coronal T2 (E, F)-weighted images reveal a large right temporo-frontal extra-axial cystic lesion of identical signal to CSF fluid in all sequences, displacing the adjacent cerebral parenchyma with mild mass effect on the midline structures. No other abnormality seen.

Diagnosis: Arachnoid Cyst

Case 108

Clinical Presentation

A 34 year-old female patient with history of epilepsy. On her past-history we note surgery for papillary carcinoma of the thyroid gland. MR Scan done to rule out brain metastasis.

Radiological Findings

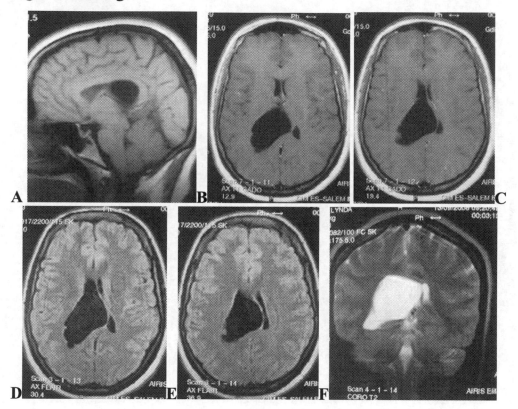

MR Scan pre-contrast sagittal (A), post-contrast axial (B, C), FLAIR (D, E) and coronal T2 (F)-weighted images showing an intra-ventricular cystic lesion enlarging the posterior part of the right lateral ventricle and presenting the same signal to CSF in all sequences except for minimal differences attributed to insulation from the normal CSF flow dynamics found within the ventricle. No contrast enhancement is seen.

Diagnosis: Intra-ventricular Arachnoid Cyst

Case 109

Clinical Presentation

A 45 year-old female patient, presented with signs of intra-cranial hypertension.

Radiological Findings

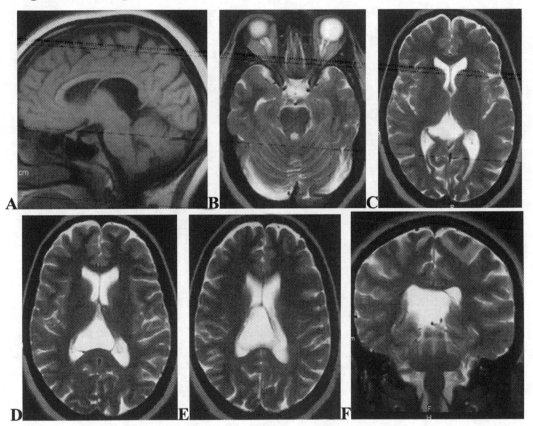

MR Scan, sagittal T1 (A), axial (B, C, D, E) and coronal (F) T2-weighted images reveal a large extra-cerebral collection in the region of quadrigeminal cistern that has similar intensity to that of ventricular fluid, being hypointense on T1 and hyperintense on T2. This cystic mass compresses mildly the posterior 3rd ventricle and upper aqueduct, which ,however remain patent as no hydrocephalus is present. Note dilated subarachnoid spaces around the optic nerfs (image B), indicating intra-cranial hypertension (usually non tumoral of idiopathic origin).

Diagnosis: Arachnoid Cyst Of Quadrigeminal Cistern

Case 110

Clinical Presentation

A 42 year-old female patient with history of chronic headaches and vertigo.

Radiological Findings

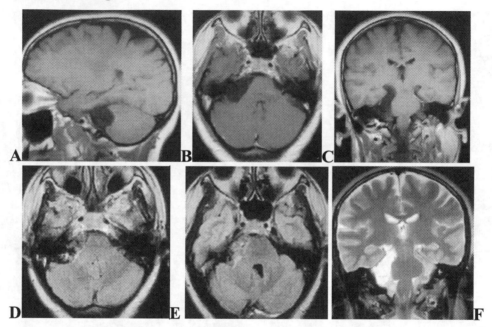

MR Scan pre-contrast sagittal (A), post-contrast axial (B) and coronal (C), axial FLAIR (D, E) and coronal T2 (F)-weighted images show a lobulated mass of the right cerebello-pontine angle extending to the ambient cistern with mass effect on the brainstem and medial temporal lobe. This mass appears of low-T1, high-T2 with heterogeneously high signal intensity on FLAIR images, indicating that the lesion is not simple arachnoid cyst but epidermoid.

Diagnosis: Epidermoid Cyst of CP Angle

Case 111

Clinical Presentation

A 31 year-old male patient, complaining of nevralgia in the territory of the right trigeminal nerve

Radiological Findings

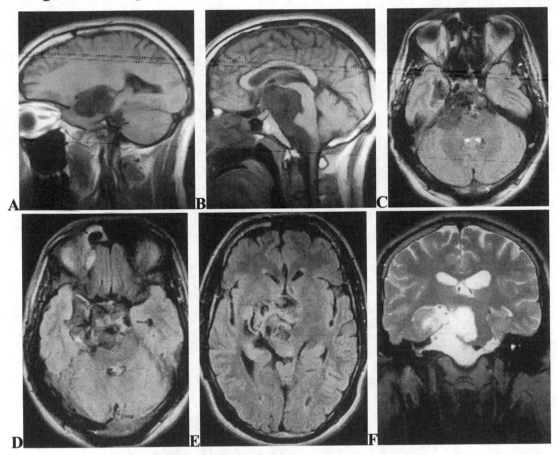

MR Scan, sagittal T1 (A, B), axial FLAIR (C, D, E) and coronal T2 (F) images demonstrate a lobulated extra-axial mass of the right internal temporal region with extension to the right cerebello-pontine and interpeduncular cisterns. This mass appears hypointense on T1 (slightly higher than CSF signal) and hyperintense on T2 with heterogeneous hypointense signal on FLAIR images. There is a significant mass effect on the cerebral peduncles, pons, pituitary stalk and optic chiasma.

Diagnosis: Temporal Epidermoid Cyst with Extension to the cerebellopontine and interpeduncular Cisterns

Case 112

Clinical Presentation

A 28 year-old female patient undergoing workup for multiple sclerosis has numbness and tingling in distal extremities.

Radiological Findings

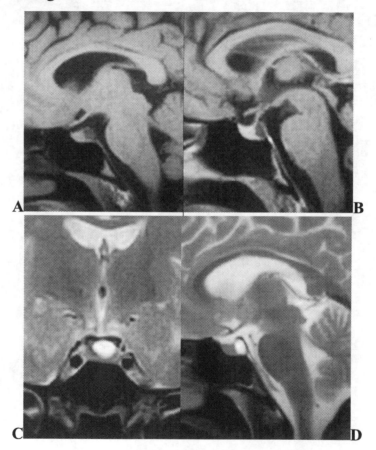

MRI Scan pre(A)-and post-contrast (B)-sagittal T1 and coronal (C)-and sagittal (D) T2-weighted images showing a small (8 mm), ovoid low-T1 and high-T2 intra-sellar mass of posterior location with supra-sellar extension, and slight mass effect on the infundibulm which is displaced anteriorly. No direct evidence of contrast enhancement.

Diagnosis: Rathke's Cleft Cyst

Case 113

Clinical Presentation

A 14 months old male child with delayed psycho-motor development. Brain CT Scan done to rule out brain malformation.

Radiological Findings

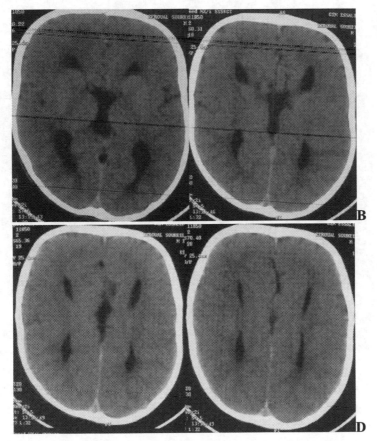

Nonenhanced Brain CT Scan showing wide separation of the lateral ventricles with straight parallel parasagittal orientation "bat-wing" appearance with absent callosal body; laterally convex frontal horns indicating absent genu of the corpus callosum; upward displacement of the 3rd ventricle in continuity with the interhemispheric fissure.

Diagnosis: Agenesis of Corpus Callosum

Case 114

Clinical Presentation

A 9 months old male child with delayed mild stone. CT done to rule out brain abnormality.

Radiological Findings

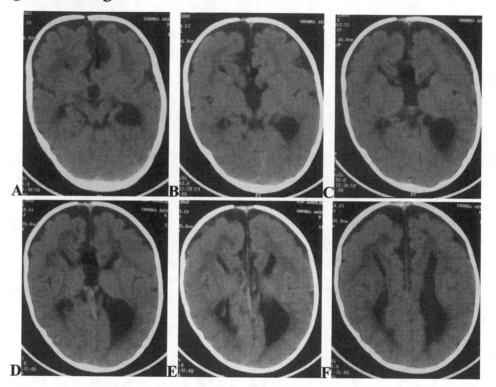

Nonenhanced Brain CT Scan reveals a wide separation of the frontal horns and lateral ventricles with upward displacement of widened 3rd ventricle "high-riding 3rd ventricle" in continuity with widened interhemispheric fissure; disproportionate enlargement of the occipital horns more on the left (colpocephaly). There is a small lesion of fatty density at the anterior interhemispheric region indicating the presence of a lipoma.

Diagnosis: Callosal Agenesis with Inter-hemispheric Lipoma

Case 115

Clinical Presentation

A female newborn, presenting abnormal movements of the extremities.

Radiological Findings

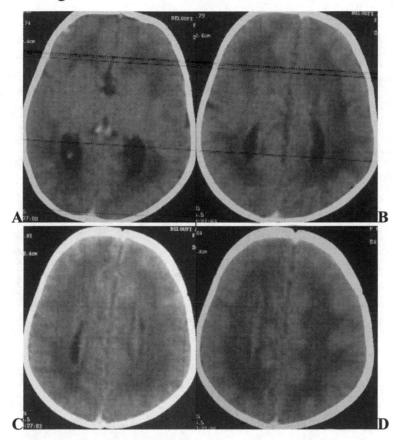

Plain brain CT Scan images demonstrate wide separation of the lateral ventricles with straight parallel parasagittal orientation "bat-wing" appearance and absent callosal body, genu and splenium with dilated occipital horns (colpocephaly). Note subependymal nodules isodense to the cortical gray matter, lining the wall of the lateral ventricles, indicating subependymal heterotopias.

Diagnosis: Callosal Agenesis with Subependymal Heterotopia

Case 116

Clinical Presentation

A 66 year-old male patient, known case of bronchial carcinoma, presenting a recent onset of headaches.

Radiological Findings

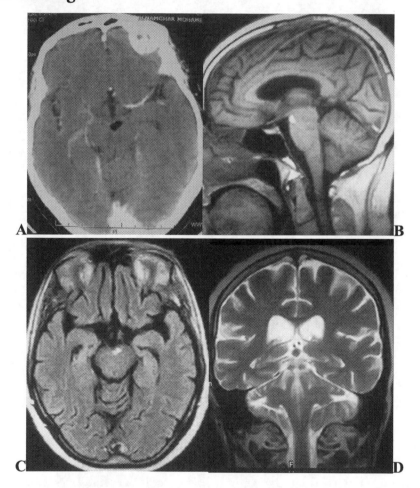

Enhanced CT Scan (A), nonenhanced MR Scan sagittal T1 (B), axial FLAIR (C) and coronal T2 (D)-weighted images demonstrate the presence of a small lesion of fatty density located in the interpeduncular cistern and appears of high signal on T1 and and FLAIR with reduced signal on T2 exactly as does the subcutaneous fat, corresponding to a lipoma (incidental finding). No cerebral metastasis seen.

Diagnosis: Lipoma of Interpeduncular Cistern

Case 117

Clinical Presentation

A 43 year-old male patient with history of chronic dorso-lumbar pain, presented for MR of spinal cord which was normal.

Radiological Findings

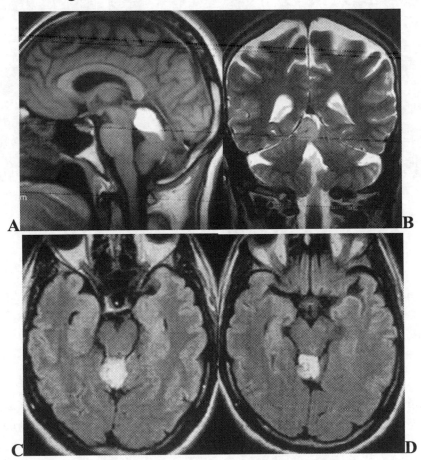

MR Scan sagittal T1 (A), coronal T2 (B) axial FLAIR (C, D) images showing an extra-axial mass filling the quadrigeminal cistern; its signal is identical to that of the subcutaneous fat on all sequences, associated with mild hypoplasia of the inferior colliculi and superior vermis. Note that the areas of signal void within the lesion may represent calcification or flow void within vessels.

Diagnosis: Quadrigeminal Cistern Lipoma (Incidental finding in this case)

Case 118

Clinical Presentation

A 6 months old female child with seizures.

Radiological Findings

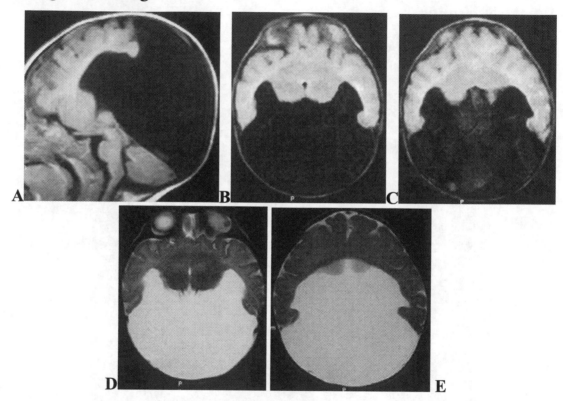

MRI Scan sagittal T1 (A), axial FLAIR (B, C) and T2 (D, E) weighted images: the sagittal T1 image shows a pancake of brain anteriorly, the holoventricle leads into a large dorsal cyst. The axial sequences (B, D) show partially fused basal ganglia and thalami with gray and white matter crossing the midline anteriorly. On image E (image slightly superior to D) shows the crescent-shaped holoventricle leading into the dorsal cyst.

Diagnosis: Alobar Holoprosencephaly

Case 119

Clinical Presentation

A child with developmental delay and seizures.

Radiological Findings

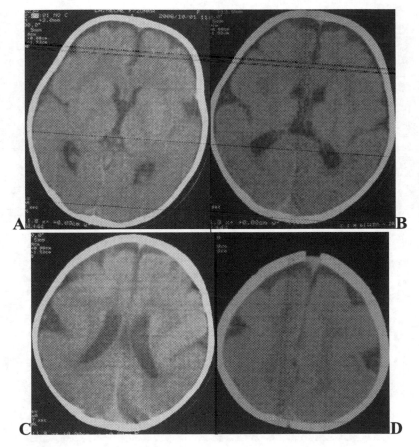

Plain brain CT Scan showing bilateral and relatively symmetrical thickened cortex with few and large gyri and shallow sulci. The sylvian fissures are abnormally vertical the lateral ventricles are mildly enlarged.

Diagnosis: Pachygyria

Case 120

Clinical Presentation

A 4 months old male child with seizures and abnormal facies.

Radiological Findings

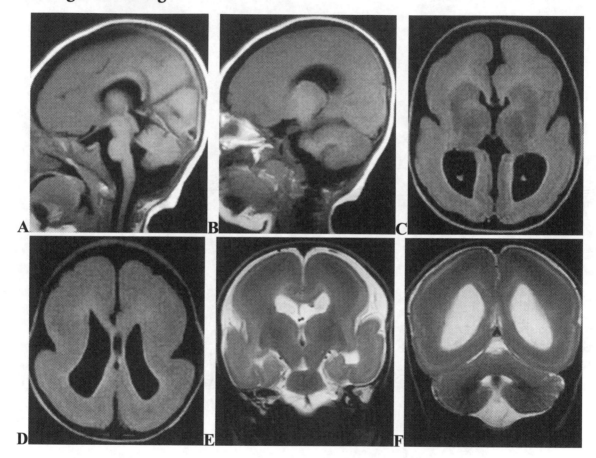

MRI Scan sagittal T1 (A, B), axial FLAIR (C, D) and cononal T2 (E, F) weighted images showing smooth brain surface and gray-white matter interface with diminished white matter, thickened cortex, shallow and vertically oriented sylvian fissures giving an "eight" appearance to the cerebrum. The corpus callosum is thinned (Callosal hypogenesis), with prominent ventricular trigones.

Diagnosis: Lissencephaly Type 1

Case 121

Clinical Presentation

A 10 year-old female child with history of epilepsy.

Radiological Findings

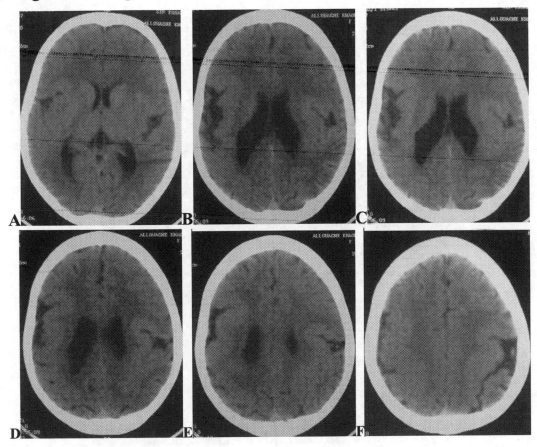

Plain brain CT Scan showing thickened insular cortex with opened and verticalized sylvian fissures, extending to the parietal lobes mainly on the right side secondary to abnormal opercularization. The enlarged ventricles are often seen in this malformation. The irregularity of the cortical-white matter junction that is also characteristic of polymicrogyria.

Diagnosis: Congenital Bilateral Perisylvian Polymicrogyria

Case 122

Clinical Presentation

A 16 months old female child with developmental delay.

Radiological Findings

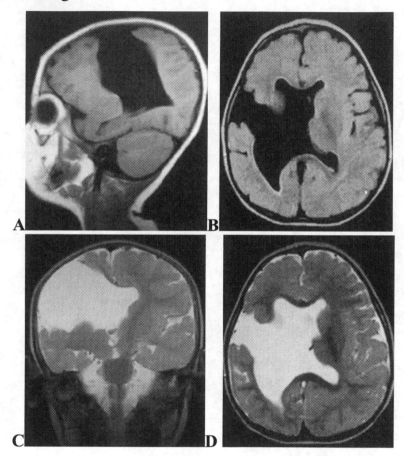

Non-Enhanced MR Scan, sagittal T1 (A), axial FLAIR (B), coronal (C) and axial (D) T2-weighted images showing a right unilateral frontotemporal cleft, surrounded by a gray matter with polymicrogyric cerebral cortex, connecting the lateral ventricles and subarachnoid CSF spaces directly through the brain parenchyma without ventricular wall or septum pellucidum.

Diagnosis: Unilateral Open Lip Schizencephaly (Type II)

Case 123

Clinical Presentation

A 9 year-old male child with history of unstable epilepsy.

Radiological Findings

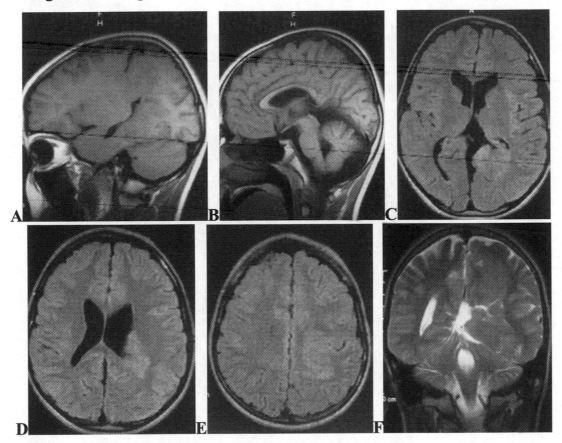

Brain MR, non-enhanced sagittal T1 (A, B), axial FLAIR (C, D,E), coronal T2 (F)-weighted images showing an isointense mass to the gray matter on all sequences, extending from the left occipital peri-ventricular white matter to the adjacent parietal cortex with mass effect on the adjacent ventricular horn. Note also the same appearance is seen in the right occipital peri-ventricular white matter but note extending to the cerebral cortex (image C). the ventricular system is relatively enlarged with dysgenesis of corpus callosum (maily the splenium).

Diagnosis: Subcortical Heterotopia with Callosal Dysgenesis

Case 124

Clinical Presentation

A 21 year-old epileptic female patient.

Radiological Findings

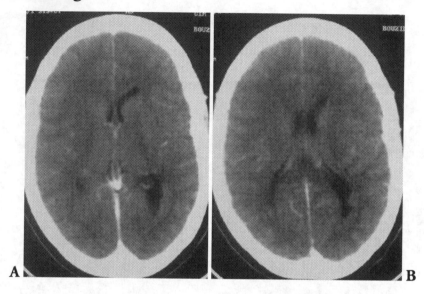

A   B

Enhanced brain CT Scan images show multiple subependymal nodular masses isodense to the cortical gray matter lining the lateral ventricles.

Diagnosis: Subependymal Grey Matter Heterotopia

Case 125

Clinical Presentation

A 10 year-old male child with temporal epileplsy.

Radiological Findings

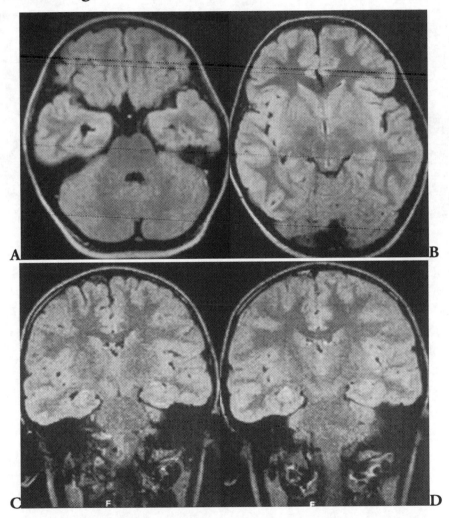

MR Scan axial (A, B) and oblique-coronal (C, D) FLAIR images showing a moderate atrophied hippocampus and parahyppocampic gyrus with dilated adjacent temporal horn. Note increased signal intensity of the right hippocampal head in comparison with the left. There is also evidence of asymmetry of tissue with loss of volume in the right hippocampus.

Diagnosis: Mesial Temporal Sclerosis (MTS)

Case 126

Clinical Presentation

A 12 year-old male child with dizziness and gait imbalance.

Radiological Findings

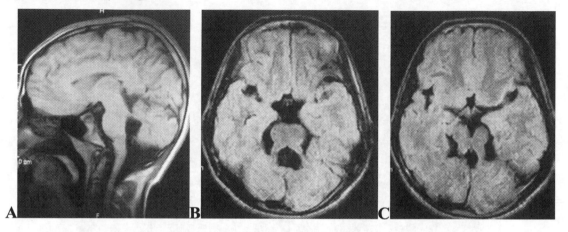

MR Scan sagittal T1 (A), axial FLAIR (B, C): Sagittal T1 image demonstrates a diminutive vermis. Axial images in particular show an enlarged fourth ventricle that is "bat-wing shaped" in configuration. The superior cerebellar peduncles are vertically oriented and elongated in the anteroposterior direction. The midbrain is small in its anteroposterior diameter, probably because of the absence of the decussation of the superior cerebellar peduncles. The characteristic appearance of the midbrain, with the enlarged superior cerebellar peduncles and the absence of their decussation has been called the "**molar tooth sign**".

Diagnosis: Joubert's Syndrome

Case 127

Clinical Presentation

A 33 year-old male patient presented with signs of increased intra-cranial pressure, static-cinetic cerebellar syndrome, pyramidal syndrome of the four limbs

Radiological Findings

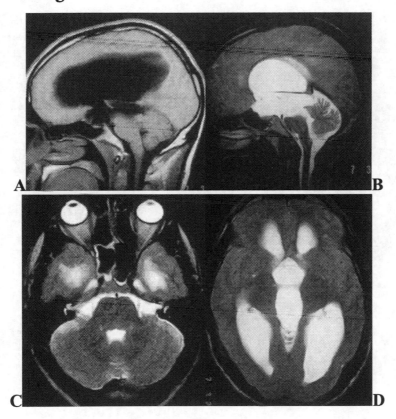

MR Scan sagittal T1 (A), sagittal (B) and axial (C, D) T2-weighted images demonstrate a cystic dilatation of the 3rd ventricle with symmetrical dilatation of the lateral ventricles and peri-ventricular interstitial edema due to transependymal resorption of CSF. Note the 4th ventricle is normal in size and shape. No mass lesion seen at the aqueduct of Sylvius.

Diagnosis: Aqueductal Stenosis

Case 128

Clinical Presentation

A 15 year-old male patient presented with cerebellar syndrome, hypotonia and extra-pyramidal signs.

Radiological Findings

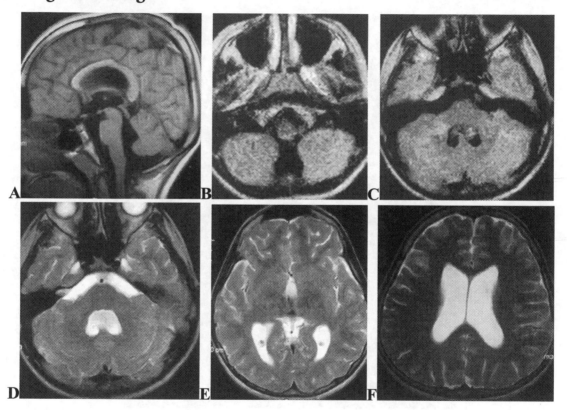

MR Scan sagittal T1 (A), axial FLAIR (B, C), and T2 (D, E, F) weighted images showing dilatation of the 4th, 3rd and lateral ventricles with no peri-ventricular interstitial edema. No intra-ventricular or intraprenchymal lesion seen.

Diagnosis: Communicating Hydrocephalus

Case 129

Clinical Presentation

A 6 months old female child with a parietal mass since birth.

Radiological Findings

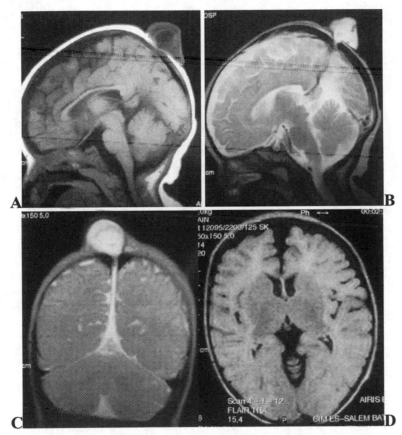

MR Scan sagittal T1 (A), sagittal and coronal T2 (B, C), and axial FLAIR (D) showing a small cystic median parietal mass of CSF signal intensity on all sequences with internal membrane (arachnoid), communicating with the peri-cerebral CSF spaces through a calvarial defect. No brain tissue seen within the cystic mass. Note the presence of a low-T1 and T2 linear structure, extending between the corpus callosum and the calvarial defect, representing most likely a rudimentary falcine sinus in an embryonic position with verticalization of the straight sinus . Otherwise benign enlargement of the subarachnoid spaces.

Diagnosis: Occipital Meningocele

Case 130

Clinical Presentation

A 21 year-old female patient with history of repeated vomiting and unsteady gait.

Radiological Findings

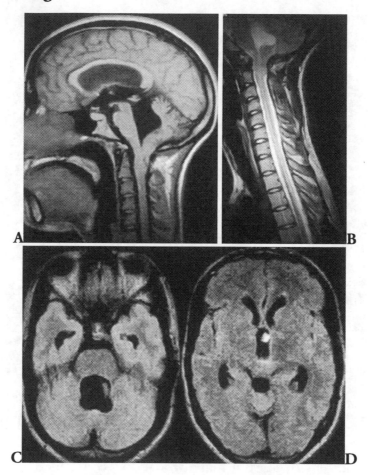

MR Scan sagittal T1 (A) and T2 (B) and axial FLAIR (C, D) images reveal a low position of the cerebellar tonsils, more than 5 mm below the foramen magnum with dilated 3rd, 4th and lateral ventricles. Note no syringohydromyelia within the cervical spinal cord.

Diagnosis: Hydrocephalus on Chiari I Malformation

Case 131

Clinical Presentation

A 5 months old male child with increased head circumference and lumbo-sacral mass.

Radiological Findings

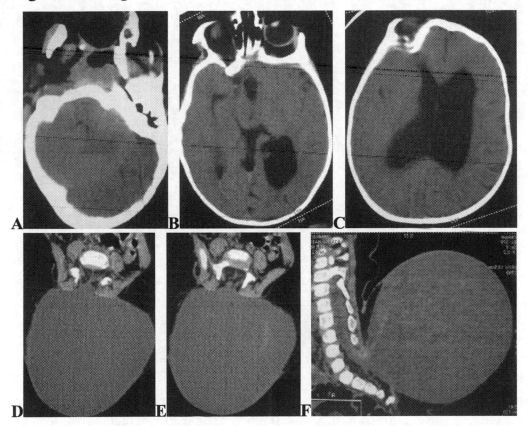

Nonenhanced CT Scan of brain (A, B, C) and spine (D, E, F): the brain CT reveals the cerebellar hemispheres extending laterally around the brainstem with obliteration of the posterior fossa cisterns and small 4th ventricle, indicating a tonsilar herniation. At supra-tentorial level there is a dilatation of the 3rd and lateral ventricles with colpocephaly and dysgenesis of the corpus callosum. The CT of spine shows a large posterior median lumbo-sacral cystic mass, communicating with the spinal canal through a defect of the posterior vertebral elements (spina bifida aperta). low position of the spinal cord with acute angulation under the last intact lamina at the upper margin of the spina bifida.

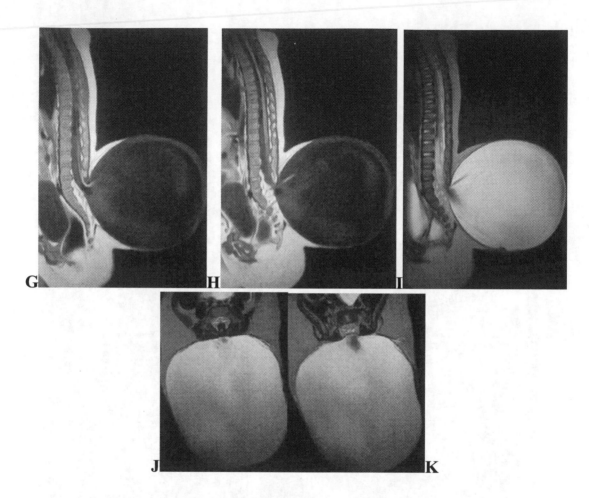

...continued, **MR Scan sagittal T1 (G, H), and sagittal and axial T2 (I, J, K)** demonstrate features characteristic of untreated myelomeningocele: dehiscence of high signal subcutaneous fat, fascia, muscle, and bone in the zone of spina bifida; low position of the spinal cord with acute angulation under the last intact lamina at the upper margin of the spina bifida; and posterior herniation of the neural tissue, forming the dorsal wall of the CSF space.

Diagnosis: Lumbo-sacral Myelomeningocele in Chiari II Maformation

Case 132

Clinical Presentation

A 15 days old newborn with an abnormally shaped head.

Radiological Findings

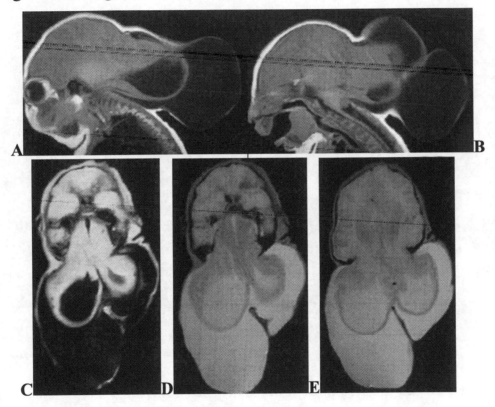

MR Scan, sagittal T1 (A, B), axial FLAIR (C), and T2 (D, E) weighted images showing a large midline occipito-parietal encephalocele through a large calvarial defect, containing both occipital lobes and a large part from the parietal lobes with dilated CSF spaces and occipital ventricular horns. The corpus callosum is absent. The posterior fossa is small in size with tonsilar herniation.

Diagnosis: Chiari III malformation

Case 133

Clinical Presentation

A 6 year-old female child with history of seizure, headache and progressive right visual deterioration. The clinical examination showing a port wine angioma involving all the right hemi-face.

Radiological Findings

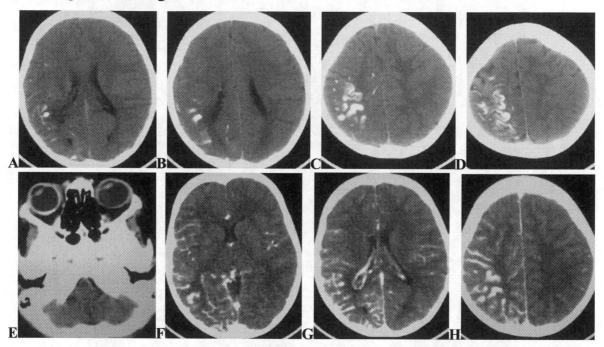

Pre-(A, B, C, D) and post-contrast (E, F, G, H) demonstrates gyriform and curvilinear calcification, most prominent in the right parietal and occipital lobes ipsilateral to the facial angioma with enlarged adjacent cerebral sulci indicating cerebral atrophy. After contrast administration there is a leptomeningeal enhancement over the right occipito-parietal region with enlargement of the right choroid plexus. Note the thickening and enhancement of the choroid of the right ocular globe indicating the presence of a choroid angioma.

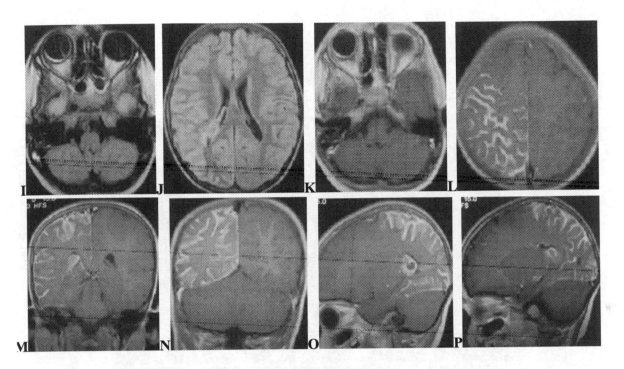

...continued, MR Scan axial FLAIR (I, J), post-contrast axial (K, L), coronal (M, N) and sagittal (O, P) T1-weighted images demonstrate FLAIR hyperintensity in the left occipito-parietal region involving cortex and subarachnoid space with no mass effect or vasogenic edema. On contrast enhanced MRI, there is enhancement within sulci in this region and asymmetric enlargement of the right choroid plexus with dilated subependymal veins. The choroid angioma of the right ocular globe is also well-visualized as arciform hyperintensity on FLAIR image (I) and thickened choroid with enhancement on post-contrast axial T1 image (K).

Diagnosis: Sturge-Weber syndrome (or Encephalotrigeminal Angiomatosis)

Case 134

Clinical Presentation

A 24 year-old female patient mentally retarded with renal failure.

Radiological Findings

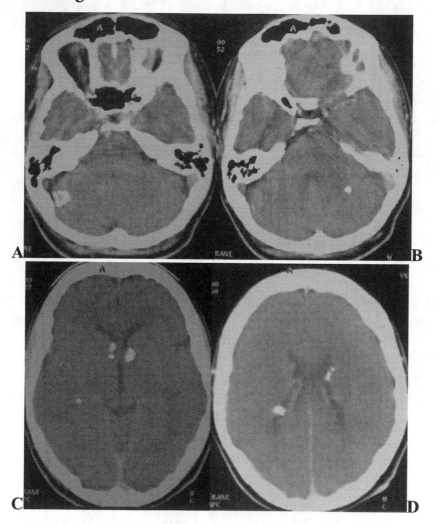

Enhanced brain CT Scan showing multiple small subependymal calcified nodules along the borders of the lateral ventricles, frontal horns and within the white matter of the cerebellar hemispheres. No other abnormality.

Diagnosis: TuberousSclerosis (Bourneville's Disease)

Case 135

Clinical Presentation

A 25 year-old male patient with seizures
.

Radiological Findings

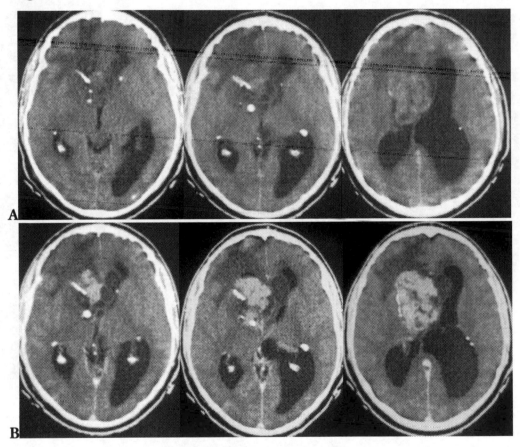

Pre(A)-and post-contrast (B) brain CT Scan Shows numerous small subependymal calcified nodules seen along the borders of the frontal horns, lateral ventricles and subcortical region, representing calcified tubers. Large right frontal tumoral mass(giant Cell Astrocytoma) of subependymal location, extending into the frontal horns with two components: solid enhanced after contrast administration filling mainly the right frontal horn, and cyst extending to the left frontal horn with large area of vasogenic edema of the right frontal lobe. Note obstructive hydrocephalus by obliteration of the foramen of Monro.

Diagnosis: Malignant Degeneration (Giant Cell Astrocytoma) with Obstructive Hydrocephalus in patient with Tuberous Sclerosis

Case 136

Clinical Presentation

A 40 year-old epileptic female patient with numerous skin café au lait spots.

Radiological Findings

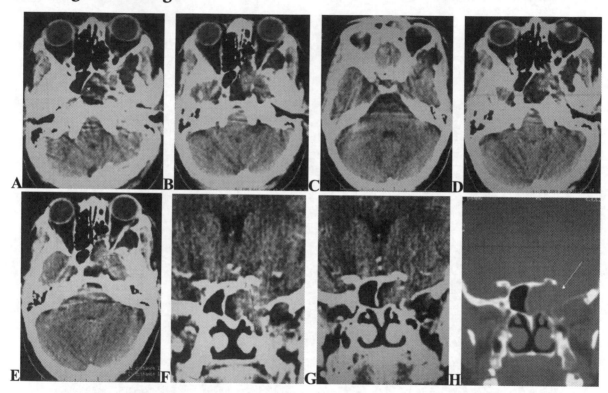

Brain CT Scan, pre-(A, B, C) and post-contrast (D, E) with coronal reconstruction (F, G) and bone settings (H) showing a soft tissue mass filling the left sphenoid sinus, presenting same density to the normal brain tissue before and after contrast administration, surrounded by area of fluid. with defect of the left lateral wall of sphenoid sinus note also the presence of a cystic structure filling the left retro-orbital space and external temporal fossa through a defect of the sphenoid wing with left axial exophthalmos grade I.

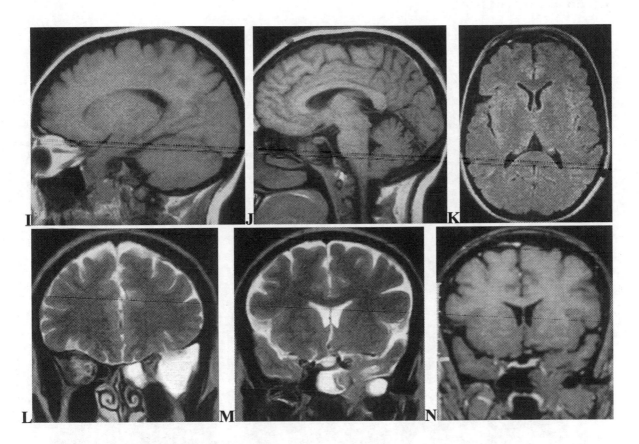

...continued, MR Scan sagittal T1 (I, J), axial FLAIR (K), coronal T2 (L, M) and post-contrast T1 (N) images confirm the herniated brain tissue from the left temporal lobe and surrounding CSF into the left sphenoid sinus, realizing an intra-sphenoid meningoencephalocele. There is a cystic mass of CSF signal in the retro-orbital space and external temporal fossa, representing a meningocele through a defect of the sphenoid wing as seen on CT Scan. Note also the presence of small subcutaneous nodules of low signal in all sequences representing neurofibromas.

Diagnosis: Von Recklinghausen's Disease (or Neurofibromatosis Type I)

Case 137

Clinical Presentation

A 16 year-old female patient, with history of bilateral hearing difficulties

Radiological Findings

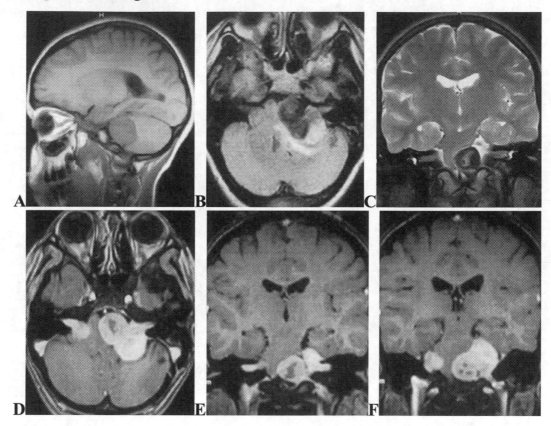

MR Scan pre-contrast sagittal T1 (A), axial FLAIR (B), coronal T2 (C) and post-contrast axial (D) and coronal (E, F) T1-weighted images showing bilateral cerebello-pontine angles masses enlarging the auditory canal with intra-canalicular extension. On the right side, the lesion appears isointense on FLAIR and T2 with intense and homogeneous enhancement after gadolinium administration, giving the appearance of a scoop of ice on a cone. On the left side the lesion is larger, lobulated, slightly hypointense on T1, heterogeneously hypointense on FLAIR and T2 with intense enhancement, except the central area which remain hypointense (necrotic area). Note mass effect on the brainstem and 4th ventricle with mild enlarged 3rd and lateral ventricles. No other cerebral lesion seen in this case.

Diagnosis: Neurofibromatosis Type 2 (or Central Neurofibromatosis)

Case 138

Clinical Presentation

A 22 year-old male patient history of chronic headaches and bilateral hearing difficulties.

Radiological Findings

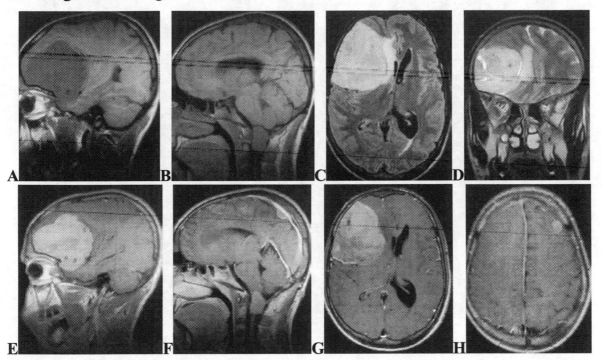

MR Scan, pre-contrast sagittal T1 (A, B), axial FLAIR (C), coronal T2 (D) and post-contrast sagittal (E, F) and axial (G, H) T1-weighted images showing multiple extra-axial lesions, the largest lesion is located in the right frontal region and appears hypointense on T1, hyperintense on FLAIR and T2 with intense and relative homogeneous enhancement after gadolinium administration, surrounded by area of vasogenic edema. The extra-axial location is evidenced by a large broad-based dural attachment and thin rim of CSF surrounding the medial margin of the lesion well-visualized on coronal T2 image. There is mass effect on the midline structures with subfalcine herniation. Two other small similar extra-axial lesions are seen, one attached to the falx cerebri (image F) and one in the left frontal region (image H). There is also an other intra-dural extra-medullary lesion of low-T1, with strong and homogeneous enhancement after contrast administration, filling the left side of the foramen magnum at the level of the bulbo-medullary junction. These lesions are typical of meningiomas.

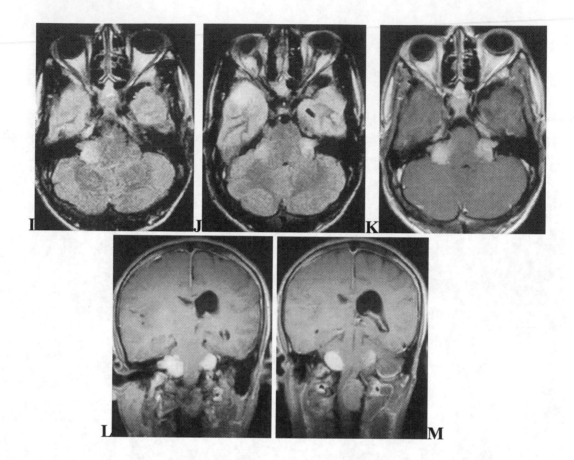

...**continued, axial FLAIR (I, J) and post-contrast axial (K) and coronal (L, M) T1-weighted images** showing bilateral cerebello-pontine angles masses enlarging the auditory canal with intra-canalicular extension. These lesions appear slightly hyperintense on FLAIR with intense and homogeneous enhancement after gadolinium administration, giving the appearance of a scoop of ice on a cone. On the right side the lesion is slightly larger (2.5 cm) than the left side (2 cm), with no significant mass effect on the brainstem or cerebellar hemispheres. Note the meningioma of foramen magnum previously described is also well-visualized on post-contrast coronal T1 (image M), compreesing and displacing the bulbo-medullary junction to the right.

Diagnosis: Neurofibromatosis Type II (or Central Neurofibromatosis)

Case 139

Clinical Presentation

A 3 year-old male child with history of recurrent otitis media, presented with swelling of the left parietal region.

Radiological Findings

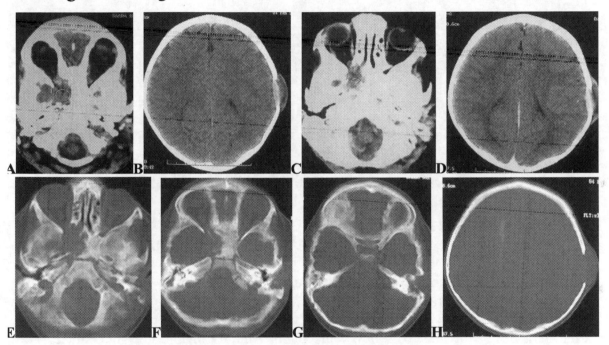

Brain CT Scan, pre-(A, B) and post-contrast (C, D) with bone settings (E, F, G, H) showing an irregular osteolytic lesion of the base of skull centered on the sphenoid (greater wing and body) with a soft tissue component which showed mild enhancement after contrast administration. Note two others similar osteolytic lesions of the petrous bones more destructive on the left side with involvement of mastoid air-cells, external and middle ears. An other similar lesion destructing the left parietal bone with a small hypodense collection and peripheral enhancement adjacent to cranial vault destruction with no intracranial extension.

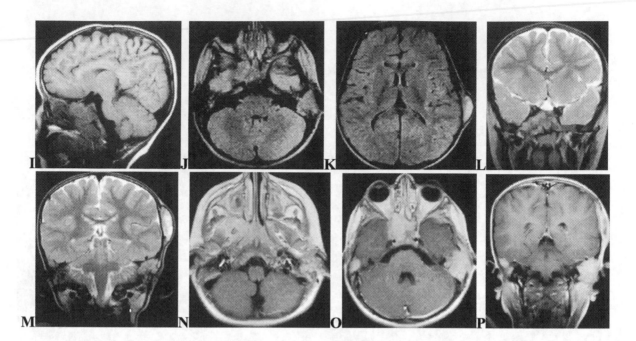

…continued, MR Scan pre-contrast sagittal T1 (I), axial FLAIR (J, K), coronal T2 (L, M) and post-contrast axial (N, O) and coronal (P)) T1-weighted images: The lesion located in the anterior base of skull appears hypointense on T1 with intermediate signal intensity on FLAIR and T2 images and shows intense enhancement after gadolinium administration. This lesion shows extension: anteriorly to the inferior orbital fissure and posterior ethmoid cells, laterally to the cavernous sinus encircling the intracavernous ICA which shows reduced caliber and finally inferiorly to the infra-temporal space infiltrating the pterygoid muscles. The lesions involving the petrous bones (external / internal ears and mastoid air-cells) show same signal intensity and enhancement as the previously described lesion. The lesion destructing the left parietal cranial vault (internal and external table) appears of high-FLAIR and T2 signal intensity with peripheral enhancement and thickening of the adjacent lepto-meningeal structures.

Diagnosis: Histiocytosis X

Spine and Spinal Cord

Tumors of Spine

Case 140

Clinical Presentation

A 37 year-old female patient presenting a flask paraplegia of progressive installation.

Radiological Findings

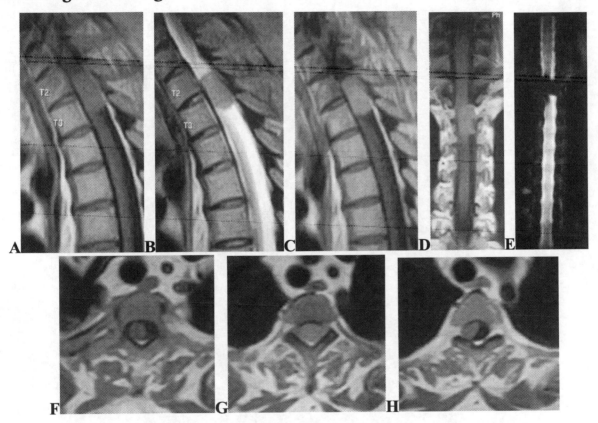

MR Scan pre -contrast sagittal T1 (A), sagittal T2 (B), post-contrast sagittal (C), coronal (D) and axial (F, G, H) and myelo-MR-2D coronal (E) showing an oval well-defined intra-dural extra-medullary lesion filling the right postero-lateral side of the spinal canal at T2-T3 level with no extension to the adjacent foramina. This lesion appears isointense to the spinal cord on T1 and T2-weighted images with intense and homogeneous enhancement after gadolinium administration. The adjacent segment of the spinal cord is severely compressed and displaced to the left side with enlargement of the subarachnoid spaces above (F) and below (H) the lesion, indicating its extra-medullary location. The myelo-MR showing a filling defect at level of the lesion, confirms the severity of compression.

Diagnosis: Thoracic Meningioma

Case 141

Clinical Presentation

A 28 year-old male patient with four months history of progressive quadriparesis.

Radiological Findings

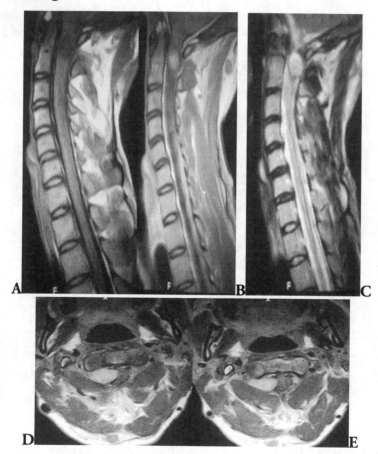

Pre-contrast sagittal T1 (A), and T2(C) and post-contrast sagittal (B) and axial (D, E) T1-weighted images showing a small, oval intra-dural extra-medullary lesion, hypointense to the spinal cord on T1 and hyperintense en T2-weighted sequence with strong and homogeneous enhancement after gadolinium administration, filling the right lateral aspect of the spinal canal at C2 level with widening of the adjacent neural foramina, compressing and displacing the spinal cord to the left side.

Diagnosis: Cervical Schwannoma

Case 142

Clinical Presentation

A 29 year-old female patient presented with history of chronic dorsal pain and radiculopathy.

Radiological Findings

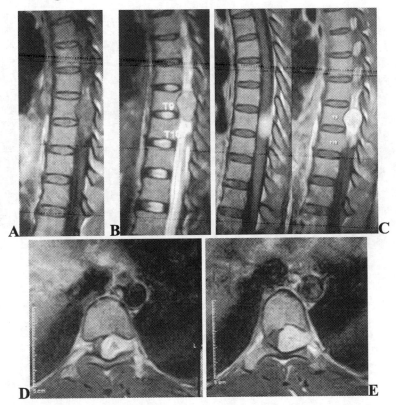

Pre-contrast sagittal T1 (A), and T2 (B) and post-contrast sagittal (C) and axial (D, E) T1-weighted images showing a small, oval intra-dural extra-medullary lesion, isointense to the spinal cord on T1 and slightly hyperintense en T2-weighted sequence with strong and homogeneous enhancement after gadolinium administration, filling the left lateral aspect of the spinal canal at T9-T10 level with widening the adjacent neural foramina, compressing the spinal cord with posterior vertebral scalloping.

Diagnosis: Dorsal Schwannoma

Case 143

Clinical Presentation

A 40 year-old female patient presented with paraparesis.

Radiological Findings

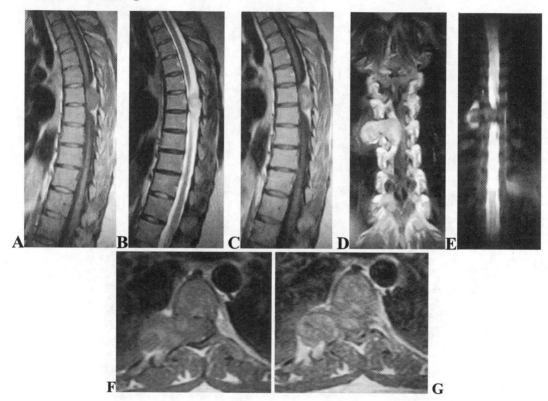

MR Scan, pre-contrast sagittal T1 (A) and T2 (B), post-contrast sagittal (C), coronal (D) and axial (F, G) T1 and coronal 2D Myelo-MR (E) images showing a small, oval intra-dural extra-medullary lesion, isointense to the spinal cord on T1 and hyperintense en T2-weighted sequence with heterogeneous enhancement after gadolinium administration, filling the right lateral aspect of the spinal canal at T6-T7 level with extra-canalar extension enlarging the adjacent neural foramina, compressing and displacing the spinal cord to the left side.

Diagnosis: Dorsal Schwannoma

Case 144

Clinical Presentation

A 37 year-old female patient with a long history of neck pain, presents with worsening symptoms.

Radiological Findings

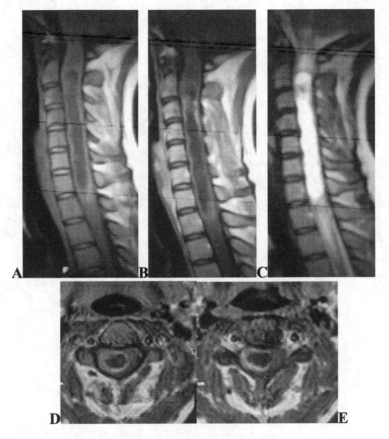

MRI Scan pre(A)-and post-contrast (B), sagittal and axial (D,E)-T1, and sagittal T2 (C)-weighted images showing an Expansile, eccentric intra-medullay mass with undulated contours, involving most of the cervical cord and medulla, presenting two components, cystic (main component) caudal with thick and irregular wall, of low-signal on T1 and high-signal on T2-weighted sequences with peripheral enhancement and mixed proximal, of isosignal on T1 and high-signal on T2-weighted sequences with nodular enhancement after contrast administration. Note localized edematous area of low-T1 and high-T2 signal intensity of the upper thoracic cord.

Diagnosis: Spinal Cord Astrocytoma

Case 145

Clinical Presentation

A 68 year-old female patient with history of radicular pain.

Radiological Findings

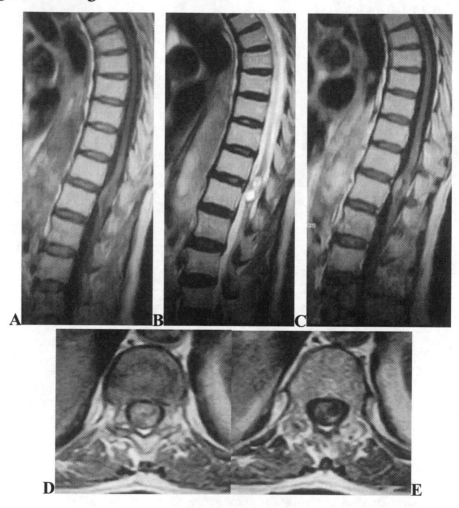

MR Scan pre(A)-and post-contrast (C) sagittal and axial (D, E) T1 and T2 (C), showing a central intra-medullary fusiform mass enlarging the spinal cord at T11-T12 level about 3 cm above the conus medullaris. This mass appears isointense to the spinal cord on T1 and T2 with central cystic areas of low-T1 and high-T2 signal. After gadolinium administration this lesion shows a herogeneous enhancement.

Diagnosis: Cord Ependymoma

Case 146

Clinical Presentation

A 60 year-old female patient presenting a progressive medullary compression syndrome with a sensitive level at T5. Past-history of breast disease.

Radiological Findings

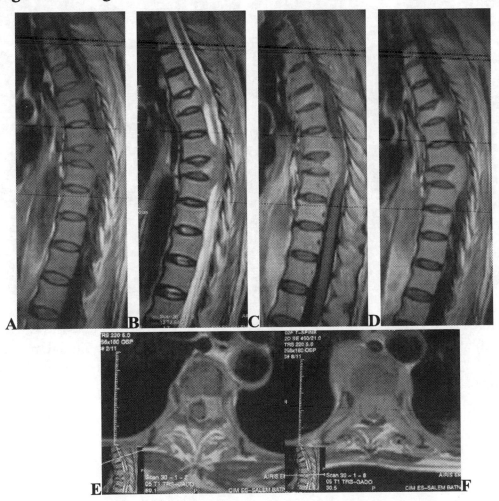

MR Scan pre(A)-and post-contrast (C, D) sagittal and axial (E, F)-T1, sagittal T2 (B) images reveal a pathologic compression-fracture of T5 and T8 vertebral bodies, which appears of low-T1 and high-T2 signal intensity with enhancement after gadolinium administration. There are pre-vertebral (at T8) and epidural (both levels) soft tissue components compressing the spinal cord mainly at T8 level.

Diagnosis: Vertebral Metastases (Breast Ca)

Case 147

Clinical Presentation

A 47 year-old female patient treated for breast Carcinoma, presented with low back pain

Radiological Findings

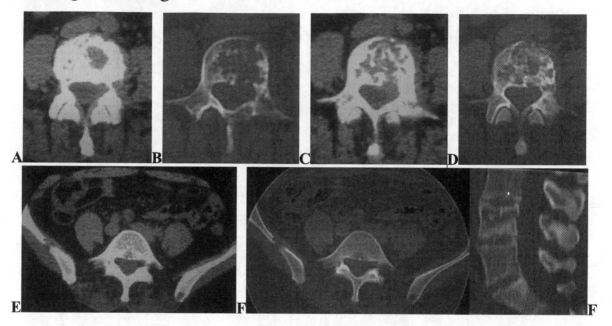

Nonenhanced CT Scan of spine showing numerous ill-defined lytic lesions, involving the L4 vertebral body and posterior arch with soft tissue density filling the epidural space mainly on the left side with right displacement of the thecal sac. Similar lytic lesions are seen in the iliac bones.

Diagnosis: Bony Metastases (from Breast Ca.)

Case 148

Clinical Presentation

A 16 year-old male patient, operated 4 years ago for ependymoma of the lower spinal cord.

Radiological Findings

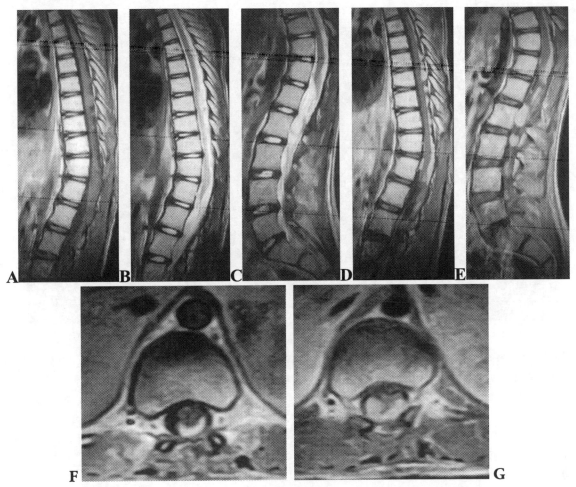

MR Scan of dorso-lumbar spine, pre(A)-and post-contrast sagittal (D, E) and axial (F, G) and sagittal T2 (B, C)-weighted images reveal multiple isointense T1 and T2 nodular lesions of various size along the dorsal surface of the spinal cord and within the thecal sac, with intense enhancement after gadolinium administration. Mild angular kyphosis at the dorsolumbar junction with laminectomy at T11, T12, L1 and soft tissues changes (past-history of surgery).

Diagnosis: Diffuse Subarachnoid Metastases (From Anaplastic Ependymoma)

Case 149

Clinical Presentation

A 44 year-old male patient, known case of acute lymphoblastic leukemia (ALL), presenting a progressive spinal cord compression.

Radiological Findings

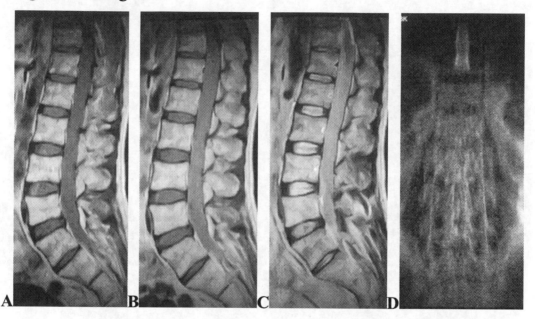

MR Scan, pre-(A) and post-contrast (B) sagittal T1, sagittal T2 (C) and coronal Myelo-MR (D) images showing patchy areas of decreased signal intensity involving the bone marrow of all vertebral bodies on both sequences, due to replacement of normal yellow marrow by tumoral cells. Note soft tissue mass filling the lumbar canal, isointense to the spinal cord on T1, slightly hyperintense on T2 with moderate enhancement after gadolinium administration, obliterating the CSF spaces and encircling the conus medullaris at T12 level as seen on T2 and Myelo-MR.

Diagnosis: Leukemic Infiltration of Vertebral Bodies and Lumbar Canal (ALL)

Case 150

Clinical Presentation

A 16 year-old female patient, presenting a progressive paraparesis with recent hypoesthesia.of the lower limbs.

Radiological Findings

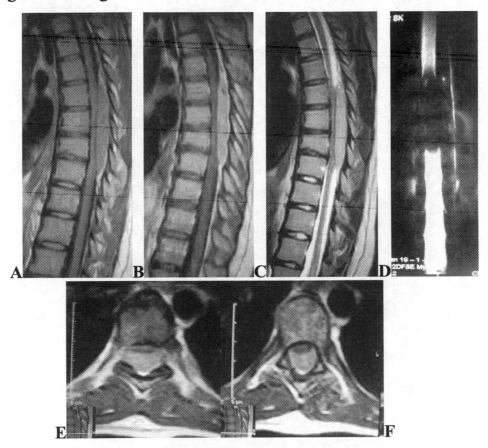

MR Scan, pre- and post-contrast sagittal (A, B), and axial (E, F) T1, sagittal T2 (C), and myelo-MR (D) show an extradural soft tissue mass dorsal to the spinal cord, isointense to the spinal cord on T1 and slightly hyperintense on T2 with mild enhancement after contrast administration, resulting in cord compression at the mid dorsal region. The Myelo-MR shows the mass as a filling defect obliterating completely the CSF spaces. The axial images showed no paraspinal component or vertebral abnormality.

Diagnosis: Peripheral Primitive Neuroectodermal Tumor (PNET)

Case 151

Clinical Presentation

A 5 year-old female child 4 months history of cervical and thoracic pain.

Radiological Findings

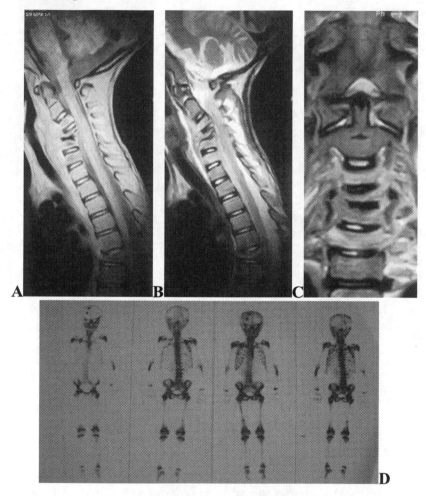

MR Scan, post-contrast sagittal T1 (A), sagittal (B) and coronal (C) T2-weighted images and whole body bone scanning with 99m-Tc-MDP (D): the MR images partial collapse of the vertebral bodies "vertebra plana" from C3 to C6 and T5 with adjacent enhancing anterior epidural soft tissue. The bone scan reveals multiple osseous areas of increased uptake involving skull, cervical and thoracic vertebra, ribs, scapula, pelvis and femoral shafts.

Diagnosis: Histiocytosis X

Case 152

Clinical Presentation

A 35 year-old female patient complaining of chronic back pain.

Radiological Findings

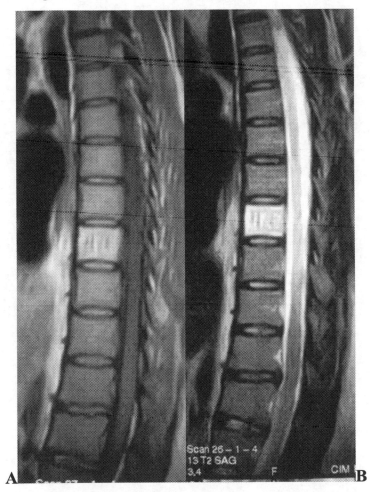

MR Scan sagittal T1 (A), and T2 (B) showing a vertical trabeculation, high-T1 and T2 (wich reflect the adipose tissue rather than the hemorrhagic component), of T8 vertebral body with no para-vertebral or epidural extension. The disc spaces are preserved.

Diagnosis: Incidental Vertebral Hemangioma

Infection of Spine

Case 153

Clinical Presentation

A 47 year-old male patient with three weeks history of neck pain, fever and progressive tetraparesis.

Radiological Findings

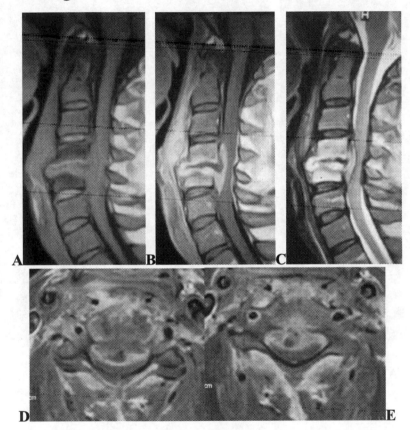

MRI Scan, pre(A)-and post(B)-contrast sagittal and axial (D, E) T1, and sagittal T2 (C) reveal a typical appearance of C4-C5 discitis and large epidural mass suggesting epidural abceess. Low-T1 and high-T2 signal intensity of C4 and C5 vertebral bodies with diffuse enhancement. Decreased height and signal intensity of C4-C5 disc with an iso-T1 and high-T2 granulation tissue in the prevertebral space, around the disc and in the anterior epidural space, forming an epidural mass compressing the adjacent portion of the spinal cord, with intense enhancement.

Diagnosis: Cervical Spondylodiscitis (Tuberculous in this case)

Case 154

Clinical Presentation

A 72 year-old male patient with severe dorsal pain.

Radiological Findings

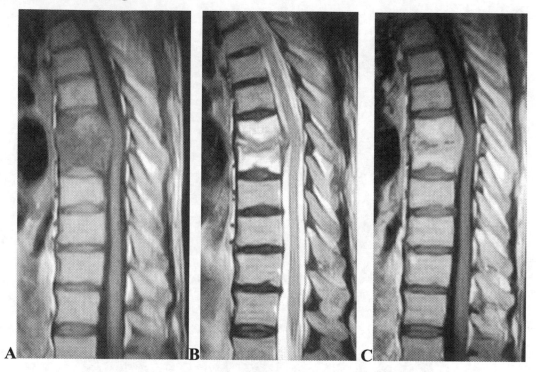

A   B   C

MR Scan, pre(A)-and post-contrast (C) sagittal T1 and sagittal T2 (B) reveal a Low-T1 and high-T2 signal intensity of T7 and T8 vertebral bodies with irregular destruction of the adjacent vertebral end-plates and disc space. After gadolinium administration there is an intense enhancement of the vertebral bodies and disc space with an epidural soft tissue component obliterating partially the pre-medullary CSF space. The spinal cord is mildly compressed with no abnormal intra-medullary signal.

Diagnosis: TB Spondylodicitis (T7-T8)

Case 155

Clinical Presentation

A 77 year-old male patient, shepherd of profession, treated for meningoencephalitis with positive serology of Wright.

Radiological Findings

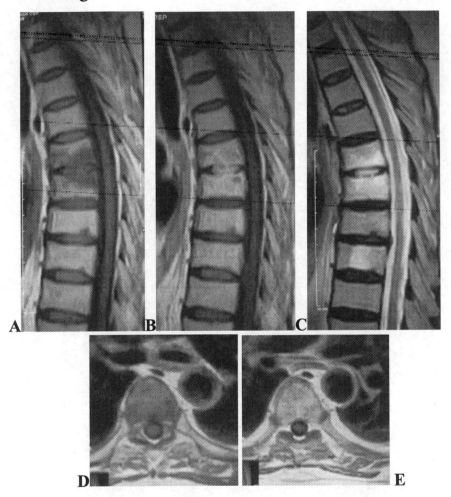

MR Scan, pre-and post-contrast sagittal (A, B) and axial (D, E) T1 and sagittal T2 (C)-weighted images showing areas of low-T1 and high T2 signal intensity of T7 and T8, affecting mainly the veretebral end-plates and intervertebral disc with significant enhancement after gadolinium administration The height of the vertebral bodies is preserved with no spinal deformities. The epidural space and the para-spinous soft tissues are not affected.

Diagnosis: Brucellar Spondylodiscitis

Case 156

Clinical Presentation

A 45 year-old male patient operated few weeks ago for L5-S1 disc prolapsed, presented with severe low back pain and fever.

Radiological Findings

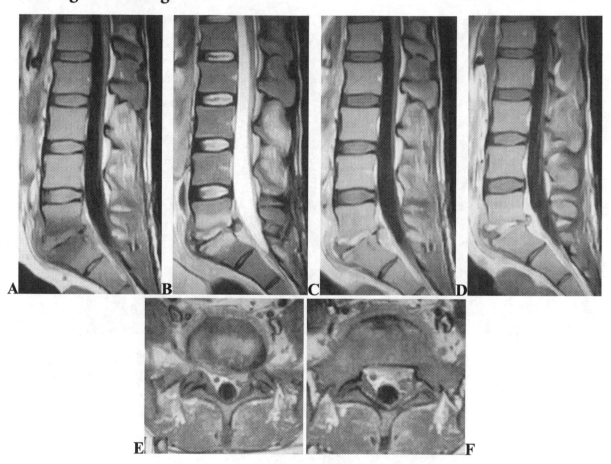

MR Scan, pre-(A) and post-contrast (C, D) sagittal T1, sagittal T2 (B) and post-contrast (E, F) axial T1 weighted images showing a low-T1 and high T2 signal intensity of L5 and S1 veretebral end-plates with irregularity and cortical destruction. After gadolinium administration there is a significant enhancement of the vertebral end-plates, within and around the disc with soft tissue thickening and enhancement at peri-vertebral and epidural spaces. Note soft tissue changes of the lumbar region (post-operative changes).

Diagnosis: Pyogenic Spondylodiscitis (staphyloccocal origin in this case)

Case 157

Clinical Presentation

A 20 year-old female patient, operated few years ago for hydatid cyst of liver. Now complaining of right radiculopathy with collapsed L5 vertebral body on lumbar x-ray.

Radiological Findings

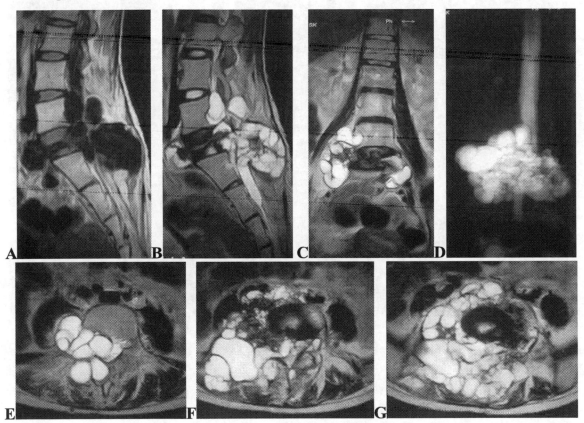

MR Scan, sagittal T1 (A), sagittal (B), coronal (B) and axial (E, F, G) T2-weighted images with Myelo-MR coronal-2D (D) reveal multiloculated cystic masses of the posterior lumbosacral soft tissues, in the territory of the posterior arch (from L4 to S1), and L5 vertebral body which is collapsed. These adjoining cystic present an intra-canalar extension from S1 up to the upper L4 vertebral end-plate with L4 posterior vertebral scalloping. There is also extension to the pre-vertebral space at L4-L5 and L5-S1 levels and to the right para-vertebral space, displacing the adjacent psoas muscle. On the myelo-MR (D) these adjoining cysts give the apearance of "bunch of grapes".

Diagnosis: Lumbo-Sacral Hydatidosis with Intra-spinal Extension

Case 158

Clinical Presentation

A 15 year-old male patient with painful scoliosis.

Radiological Findings

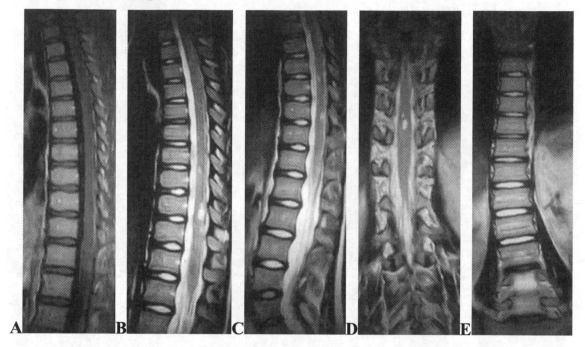

MR Scan post-contrast sagittal T1 (A), sagittal (B, C) and coronal T2 (D, E)-weighted images reveal a diffuse irregular leptomeningeal enhancement that fill the entire subarachnoid space along the dorsal spinal cord **(A)**. Indistinct poorly defined posterior margin of the spinal cord due to thickened inflammatory leptomeningeal structures with small high signal intensity intra-medullary lesions involving the mid and lower spinal cord indicating associated myelitis **(B, C, D)**. Lumbar scoliosis of right sided convexity **(E)**.

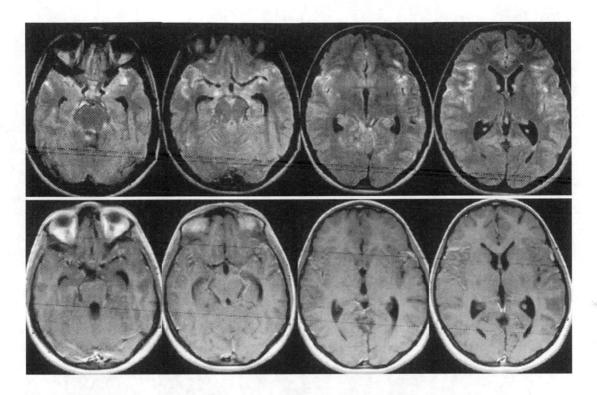

...continued. Post-contrast FLAIR (1st row) and T1-weighted images (2nd row) show a thick nodular enhancement of the basal cisterns around the middle cerebral arteries, sylvian fissures and cerebral sulci with raised intracranial pressure as indicated by the mild dilatation of the ventricular system due to obstruction in the CSF flow.

Diagnosis: Tuberculous Arachnoiditis (Brain & Spine) with Myelitis

Case 159

Clinical Presentation

A 42 year-old female patient with abrupt onset of tetraplegia and sensitive level at the nipples. Non-specific changes on blood and CSF tests.

Radiological Findings

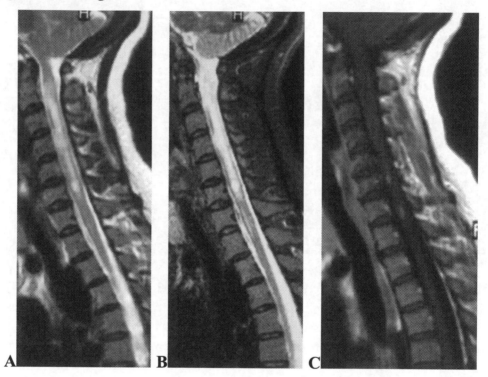

MRI Scan sagittal T2 (A, B) and post-contrast sagittal T1 (C)-weighted images: The sagittal weighted images show a swelling of the cervical spinal cord with multiple areas of high signal intensity separated by skip areas of normal cord. This appearance is against the diagnosis of a neoplasm. The post-gadolinium sagittal T1-weighted image shows small nodular areas of enhancement and also a patchy enhancement of both sides of the upper cord.

Diagnosis: Acute Transverse Myelitis

Case 160

Clinical Presentation

A 13 year-old male child presented with abrupt onset of tetraplegia, abolished osteo-tendinous reflexes, neurovegetatives and sphincterian disorders. Non specific changes on blood and CSF tests. No history of recent viral illness.

Radiological Findings

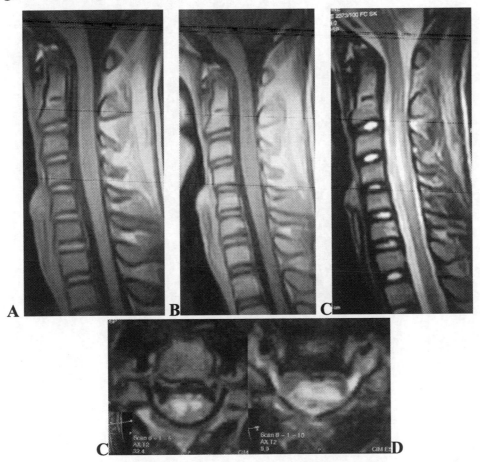

MR Scan, pre-(A) and post-(B) contrast sagittal T1 and sagittal (C) and axial (D, E) T2-weighted images show a swelling of the spinal cord extending from C2-C3 up to C5-C6 level with intra-medullary hyperintensity on T2 images affecting mainly the central portion of the spinal cord. On post-contrast sagittal T1 there is no evidence of blood-brain barrier disruption.

Diagnosis: Acute Transverse Myelitis

Case 161

Clinical Presentation

A 22 year-old male patient electrocuted during an attack in the dorsal region, presented with dorsal wound and paraplegia.

Radiological Findings

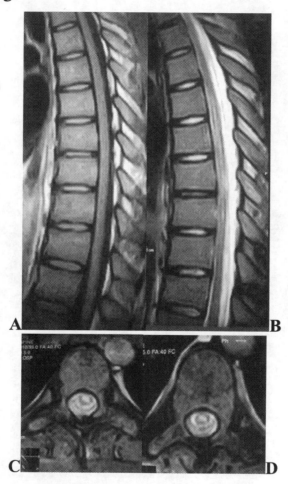

MR Scan sagittal T1 (A) and sagittal (B)and axial (C, D) T2-weighted images showing hyperintensities of the thoracic spinal cord on T2 (with no abnormality shown on T1), extending down into the conus, of anterior location on the axial images, indicating ischemic changes within the cord according to the clinical history.

Diagnosis: Ischemic Myelopathy

Degenerative and Trauma. of spine

Case 162

Clinical Presentation

A 53 year-old male patient with right C6 radiculopathy.

Radiological Findings

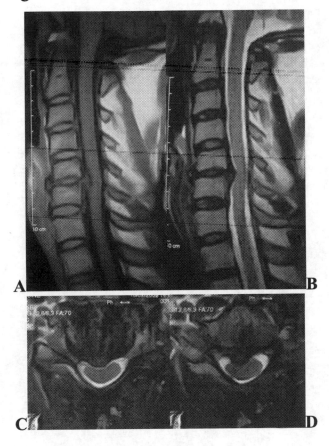

MR Scan, sagittal T1 (A), T2 (B) and axial T2 (C, D) images showing a loss of the normal height of C5-C6 intervertebral disc with a huge right para-median disc herniation, obliterating the anterior CSF space, compressing the anterior aspect of the cord and the emergence of C6 ventral root. No abnormal signal within the spinal cord.

Diagnosis: Cervical Disc Herniation

Case 163

Clinical Presentation

A 48 year-old male patient, presenting a pyramidal syndrome of the four limbs

Radiological Findings

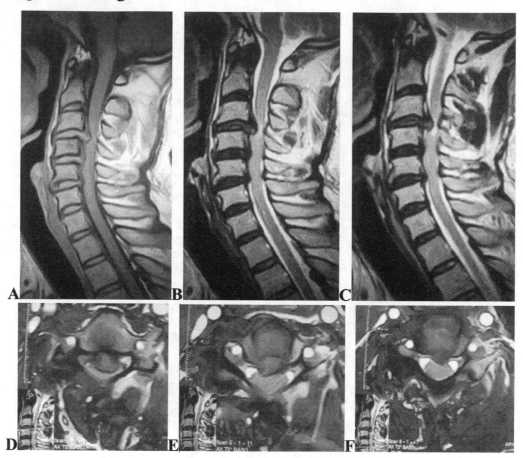

MR Scan, sagittal T1 (A), T2 (B, C) and axial T2 (D, E, F) images: Decreased height and signal intensity of C3-C4 intervertebral disc with a huge central disc herniation, effacing the anterior CSF space and compressing severely the spinal cord which appears atrophied with area of high signal intensity on T2 images (myelomalacia or gliosis). Decreased height and signal intensity of C4-C5 and C5-C5 intervertebral discs with disc herniation at both levels, right para-median at C4-C5 and left para-median at C5-C6, effacing the anterior CSF space and compressing the spinal cord.

Diagnosis: Triple Cervical Disc Prolapse with Myelopathy

Case 164

Clinical Presentation

A 52 year-old male patient presenting a paraparesis of the lower limbs.

Radiological Findings

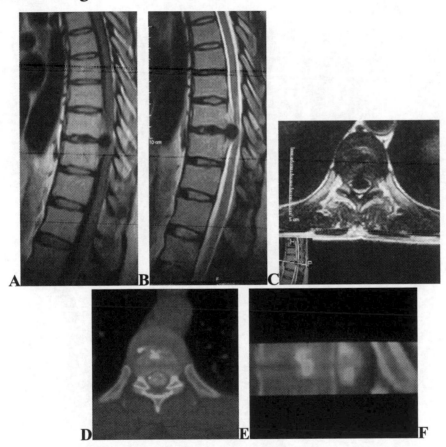

MR Scan, sagittal T1 (A) , sagittal (B) and axial (B) T2, axial CT Scan at T9-T10 level (D) with sagittal reconstruction (E) showing decreased height and signal intensity of T9-T10 intervertebral disc with posterior central hypointense (calcified) disc prolapsed, obliterating the anterior subarachnoid space and compressing severely the adjacent segment of spinal cord. Note a granulation tissue filling partially the anterior epidural space around the discal fragment. CT Scan demonstrates well the calcified disc prolapsed and Schmorl's nodes of the vertebral end-plates.

Diagnosis: Calcified Dorsal Disc Proplapse

Case 165

Clinical Presentation

A 32 year-old female patient with long-standing history of backache radiating to the right lower limb.

Radiological Findings

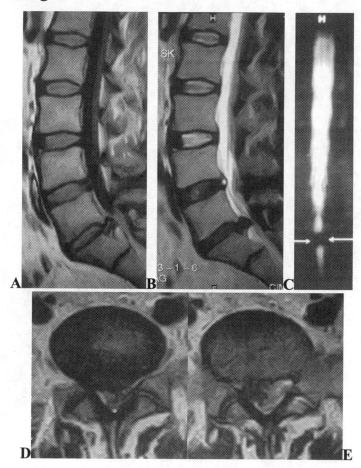

MRI Scan, sagittal T1 (A), T2 (B), coronal myelo-MRI (C) and axial T2 (C): Decreased height and signal intensity of L5-S1 intervertebral disc with huge right postero-lateral disc herniation, filling partially the anterior epidural space, compressing the thecal sac and adjacent S1 nerve root. The myelo-MRI demonstrates the degree of compression of the thecal sac and its content"arrows".

Diagnosis: Disc Herniation

Case 166

Clinical Presentation

A 38 year-old male patient complaining of left radiculopathy.

Radiological Findings

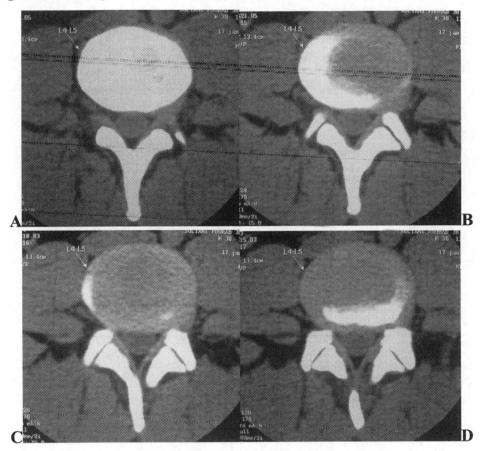

Lumbar CT Scan at L4-L5 level showing a left foraminal disc herniation, obliterating the neural foramina, compressing and displacing the adjacent L4 nerve root.

Diagnosis: Left Foraminal Disc Herniation at L4-L5

Case 167

Clinical Presentation

A 40 year-old female patient, complaining of chronic low back pain.

Radiological Findings

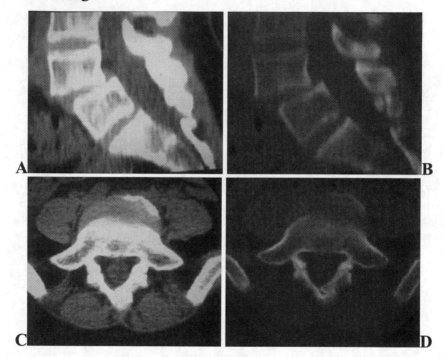

CT Scan of lumbo-sacral region sagittal reconstruction with bone settings (A, B) and axial cuts with bone settings at L5-S1 level (C, D) showing a spondylolisthesis grade I of L4 on L5 by bilateral spondylolysis seen as a bilateral defect of the neural arch or lysis of the pars interarticularis. Note the presence of transitional abnormality with sacralisation of L5 and spina bifida occulta.

Diagnosis: Spondylolisthesis by bilateral Spondylolysis

Case 168

Clinical Presentation

A 55 year-old female patient complaining of chronic low back pain.

Radiological Findings

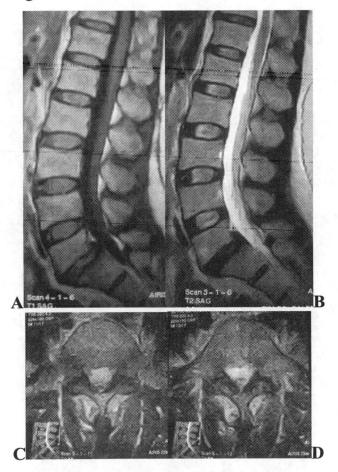

MR Scan sagittal T1 (A) and T2 (B) and axial T2 (C, D) showing a spondylolisthesis grade I of L5 on S1 by bilateral spondylolysis as seen on axial images. Note decreased height and signal intensity of L5-S1 intervertebral disc with irregularity and high T1 and T2 signal intensity of the vertebral end-plates indicating a degenerative discogenic disease grade II.

Diagnosis: Spondylolisthesis of L5 on S1 by Bilateral Spondylolysis

Case 169

Clinical Presentation

A 60 year-old female patient, presenting a queue de cheval syndrome after rachianesthesia 2 months ago for biopsy of an endometrial tumor.

Radiological Findings

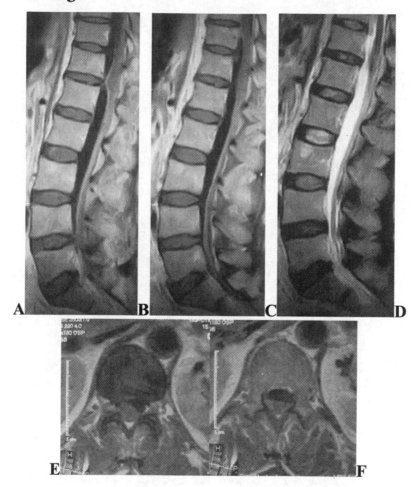

MR Scan, post-contrast sagittal (A, B) and axial (E, F) T1 and sagittal T2 (D)-weighted images showing a biloculated fusiform anterior subdural collection of CSF signal intensity, extending from T10 up to L5 with thin posterior enhancement, compressing and displacing the conus medullaris and dural sac posteriorly. No abnormal signal seen within the lower spinal cord.

Diagnosis: Subarachnoid Hygroma

Case 170

Clinical Presentation

A 33 year-old male patient involved in RTA few days ago, presenting an areflexic right monoparesis.

Radiological Findings

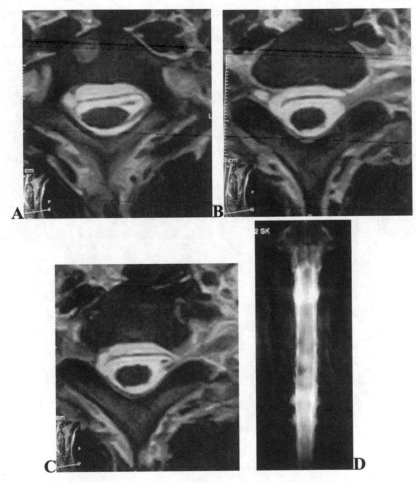

MR Scan of cervical region, axial T2-weighted images at C6-C7 (A, B) and C7-C8 (C) with coronal Myelo-MR (D) show no right ventral nerve root at C6-C7 and C7-C8 levels with evidence of pseudomeningocele at both level well-visualized on the coronal Myelo-MR, indicating nerve roots avulsion.

Diagnosis: Avulsion of the right C7 and C8 Nerve Roots

Case 171

Clinical Presentation

A 40 year-old male patient involved in RTA, presented with paraplegia with no sensitive disorder.

Radiological Findings

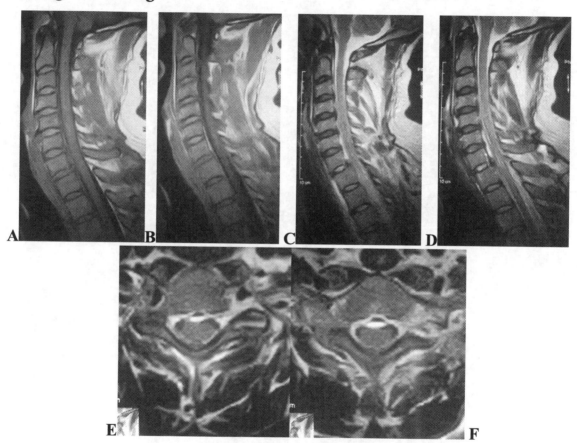

MR Scan, sagittal T1 (A, B), T2 (C,D) and axial T2 (E, F) weighted images showing C7-T1 subluxation with localized rupture of the posterior common vertebral ligament (PCVL) and small non-compressive epidural hematoma of high T1 and T2 signal intensity posterior to C6 /C7 vertebral bodies. Note small localized intra-medullary high-T2 signal area at the level of C7-T1 corresponding to a focal area of edematous contusion. Widening of C7-T1 interspinous space with area of high signal intensity indicating ligamentous injury.

Diagnosis: C7-T1 Subluxation with Spinal Cord, PCVL and Interspinous ligament Injuries

Case 172

Clinical Presentation

A 24 year-old female patient, victim of knife attack with numerous wounds in the posterior and left lateral area of the neck. The clinical examination reveals a monoparesis of the left upper limb.

Radiological Findings

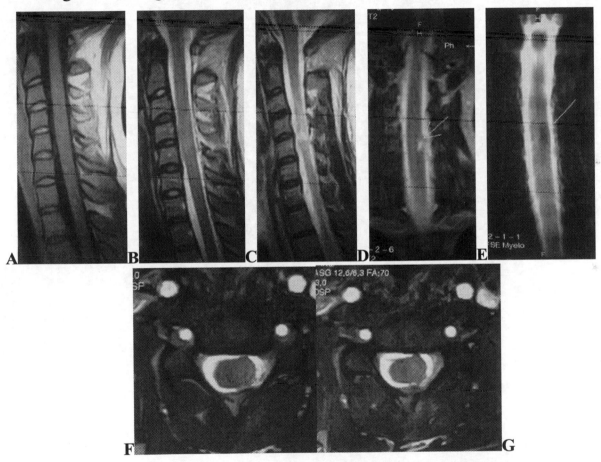

MR Scan, Sagittal T1 (A), sagittal and coronal T2 (B, C, D), coronal myel-MR (E) and axial T*2-BASG (E, F): showing a localized swelling of the spinal cord at C4-C5 level, obliterating the adjacent anterior CSF space with focal intra-medullary high-T2 signal intensity area, located on the left side at the emergence of the ventral C5 nerve root, representing an edematous contusion. No other abnormatity

Diagnosis: Spinal Cord Injury

Case 173

Clinical Presentation

An 18 year-old patient involved in road traffic accident, presenting paraplegia with T6 sensitive level.

Radiological Findings

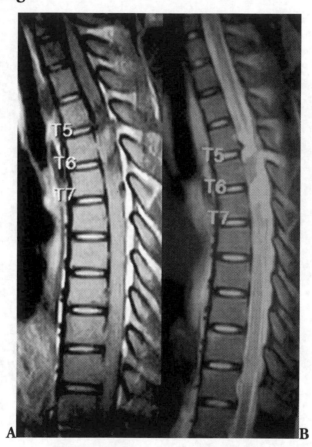

MRI Scan sagittal T1 (A) and T2 (B)-weighted images demonstrate a swelling of the spinal cord from T5 to T7 level with long segment of signal abnormality extending from T4 up to T7 of low-T1 and high-T2 (spinal cord edema and contusion), separated by skip area of normal cord at T6 level. The ligamentum flava is ruptured at T5-T6. No other ligamentous injury is demonstrated. Normal signal intensity of the marrow of the vertebral bodies.

Diagnosis: Spinal Cord Injury

Case 174

Clinical Presentation

A 56 year-old paraplegic male patient with history of RTA 3 years ago.

Radiological Findings

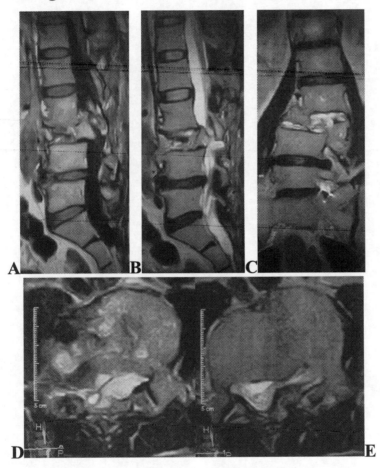

MR Scan sagittal T1 (A), sagittal (B), coronal (C) and axial (D, E) T2-weighted images showing a compression-fracture of L3 vertebral body with numerous fragments displaced anteriorly, laterally and posteriorly, the lastest one fills the epidural space and compresses the thecal sac with the fragment from the right pedicle. The coronal image shows the lateral translation of the spine indicating a dislocation. On axial images the inferior L3 end-plate lies anterior to the superior L4 end-plate.

Diagnosis: Compression-Fracture of L3 with Lateral Dislocation of Spine

Malformations of Spine

Case 175

Clinical Presentation

A 10 year-old female child with urinary incontinence, renal ectopia and an abnormal facies.

Radiological Findings

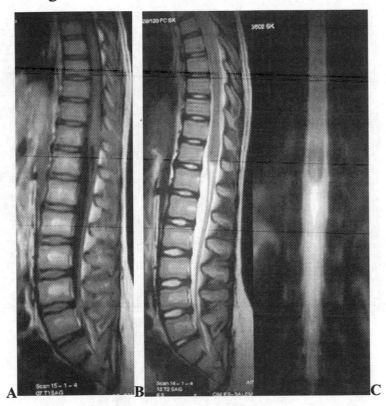

MR Scan sagittal T1 (A), T2 (B) weighted images and coronal 2D myelo-MR (C), show that the conus terminus is blunted, ending at T11 level. The spinal column is normal except for the sacrum, S2 an S3 are dysplastic and the S4, S5 segments and the coccyx are absent.

Diagnosis: Caudal Regression Syndrome

Case 176

Clinical Presentation

A 9 year-old male child with history of acute paraplegia and sphinterian disorders.

Radiological Findings

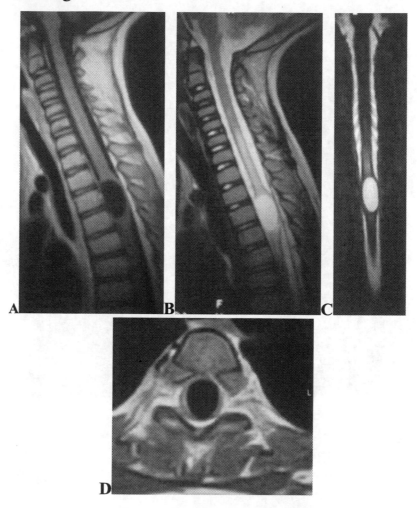

MRI Scan, pre-contrast sagittal T1 (A), T2 (B), coronal 2D myelo-MRI (C) and post-contrast axial T1(D)-weighted images demonstrate a Low-T1 and high-T2 well-defined, oval intra-medullary cystic lesion enlarging the spinal cord at the level of T3-T4. No soft tissue component or abnormal enhancement after gadolinium administration. The spinal cord above and below the lesion shows an abnormal high-T2 areas consisting of myelopathy.

Diagnosis: Intra-Medullary Cystic Lesion 'Focal Syrinx' with myelopathy

Case 177

Clinical Presentation

A 32 year-old female patient with statico-cinetic cerebellar syndrome, central vestibular syndrome, and bilateral irritative pyramidal syndrome.

Radiological Findings

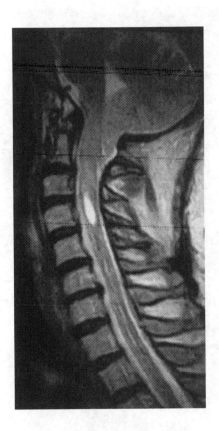

MRI Scan Sagittal T2-weighted image shows a herniation of the cerebellar tonsils below the foramen magnum. The cerebellar tonsils are abnormally beaked with reduced amount of cerebrospinal fluid surrounding the foramen magnum and obliteration of cisterna magna. The 4th ventricle and lateral ventricles (not shown) are dilated indicating obstructive hydrocephalus. There is a small, oval, high-T2 spinal cord hydrosyringomyelia at C3-C4 level.

Diagnosis: Chiari I Malformation with Hydrocephalus and Cervical Cord Hydrosyringomyelia

Case 178

Clinical Presentation

40 year-old male patient with lombosacral mass since birth.

Radiological Findings

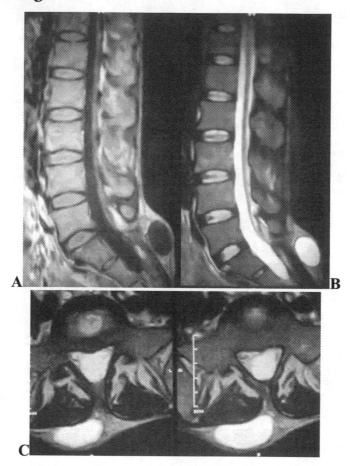

MRI Scan sagittal T1 (A), T2 (B) and axial T2 (C)-weighted images reveal a widening of the lower dural sac with thin, elongated spinal cord extending all the way down to L5-S1 level with acute angulation of the cord under the last intact lamina at the upper margin of the spina bifida. Large ovoid sacral cystic mass with thin and regular wall, located in the subcutaneous tissue following the CSF signal intensity on T1 and T2, communicating with the dural sac through the defect of the posterior elements of S1 (spina bifia).

Diagnosis: Tethered Spinal Cord with Sacral Myelomeningocele

Case 179

Clinical Presentation

A 12 year-old male child with congenital elevated left scapula. MR done to rule out vertebral anomalies.

Radiological Findings

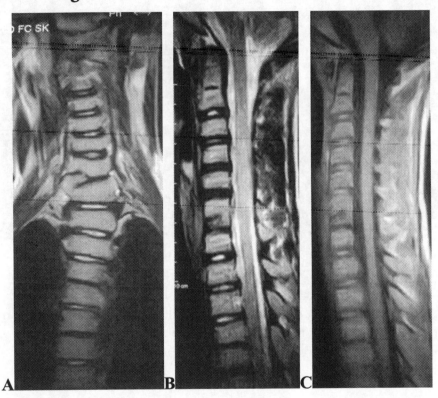

MR Scan coronal and sagittal T2 (A, B) and sagittal T1 (C)-weighted images showing a cervico-dorsal scoliosis of left sided convexity centered on a vertebral abnormality as a right hemi-vertebrae inserted between C6 and C7 vertebral bodies, partially fused with the right side of C7.

Diagnosis: Congenital Cervico-dorsal Scoliosis on vertebral abnormality

Case 180

Clinical Presentation

A 11 year-old female patient with lumbar spine deformity.

Radiological Findings

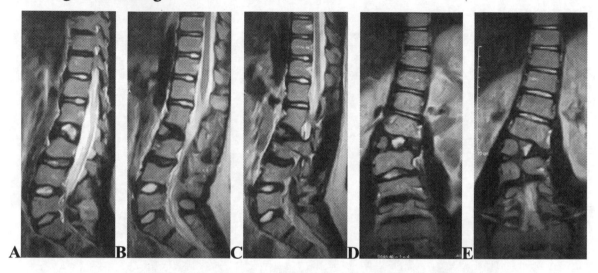

MR Scan sagittal (A, B, C) and coronal (D, E) T2-weighted images reveal a lumbar scoliosis of right sided convexity with anomalies of the vertebral segmentation which appear as sagittal cleavage of L2 and L3 vertebral bodies well-visualized on coronal images and giving the appearance of butterfly wings vertebrae.

Diagnosis: Malformative Scoliosis

Case 181

Clinical Presentation

A 62 year-old male patient with paraparesis and sensitive level at L1.

Radiological Presentation

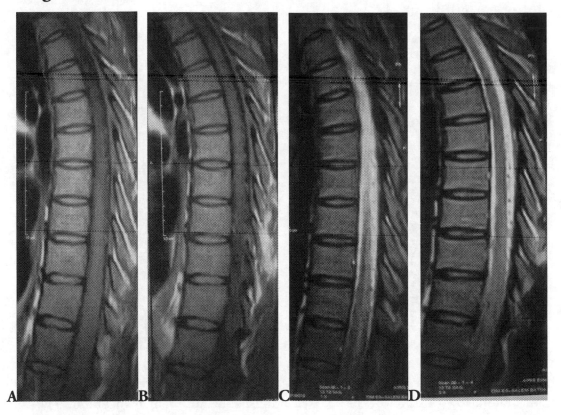

MR Scan sagittal T1 (A, B) and T2 (C, D)-weighted images showing multiple serpiginous extramedullary flow void structures along the dorsal surface of the mid and lower dorsal spinal cord, representing abnormal dilated pial veins with increased intrinsic cord signal at same level on T2-weighted image. Mild anterior displacement of the adjacent spinal cord.

Diagnosis: Spinal Dural Arteriovenous Fistula (SDAVF)

Case 182

Clinical Presentation

A 27 year-old male patient with long history of neck pain. The radiographs of the cervical spine show numerous vertebral blocks.

Radiological Findings

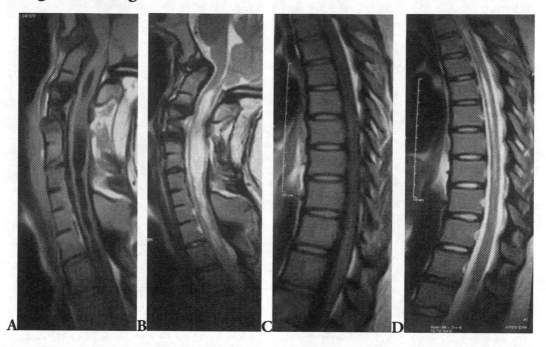

MR Scan, sagittal T1 and T2 images of cervical (A, B) and dorsal (C, D) spine demonstrate a low position of the cerebellar tonsils in the foramen magnum. The spinal cord is enlarged especially in its cervical segment, due to the presence of an intra-medullary cystic lesion with lobulated contours, of low-T1 and high-T2 signal intensity, extending from the bulbo-medullary junction up to T9 level. There are multiple vertebral blocks extending from C2-C3 up to T3-T4 level. The odontoid process shows an upward displacement (more than 7 mm) above Chamberlain line indicating basilar invagination; it shows also posterior angulation with increased basal angle indicating platybasia.

Diagnosis: Chiari I Malformation with Hydrosyringomyelia, Vertebral Blocks, Basilar Invagination and Platybasia

Case 183

Clinical Presentation

A 60 year-old male patient with past-history of surgery for disc prolapsed at L4-L5, complaining of weakness of the lower limbs.

Radiological Findings

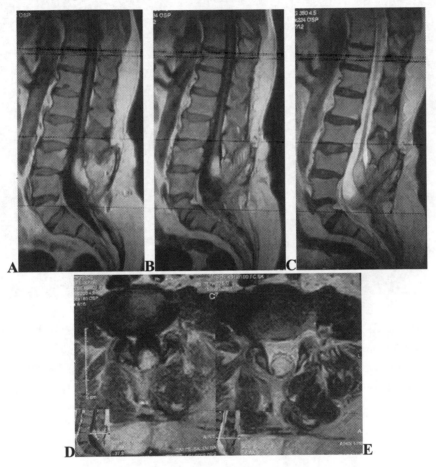

MR Scan, sagittal T1 (A, B), sagittal and axial T2 (C, D, E) images reveal a low position of the conus medullaris at L3-L4 level, fixed by a well-defined fusiform intra-canalar lipoma of high signal on T1, with mild attenuation of the signal on T2-weighted images as does the subcutaneous fat. The ventral subarachnoid space is enlarged. The posterior vertebral elements are intact except the area of laminectomy with fibrotic changes of the posterior soft tissue.

Diagnosis: Tethered Spinal Cord Fixed By a Lipoma

Case 184

Clinical Presentation

A 20 year-old male patient with long history of lower limbs weakness.

Radiological Findings

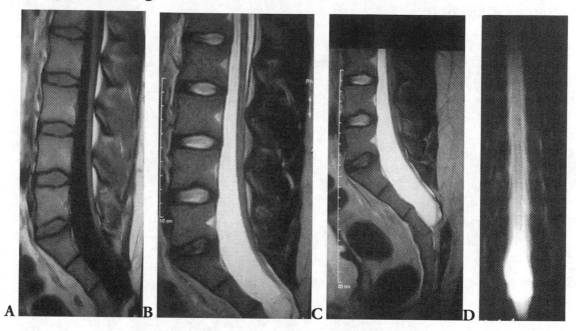

MR Scan, sagittal T1 (A), and T2 (B, C) and coronal 2D myelo-MR (D) images showing a thin, elongated spinal cord extending all the way down to the sacral level with anterior angulation, adherent to a small intraspinal lipoma, well-visualized on Sagittal T1 image as high signal mass at S4 level. There is a spina bifida occulta S2 and S3 with enlarged anterior lumbo-sacral subarachnoid space.

Diagnosis: Tethered Spinal Cord with Terminal Spinal Lipoma

Case 185

Clinical Presentation

A 15 year-old female patient, complaining of chronic low back pain and lower limbs weakness. No history of spinal traumatism or infection.

Radiological Findings

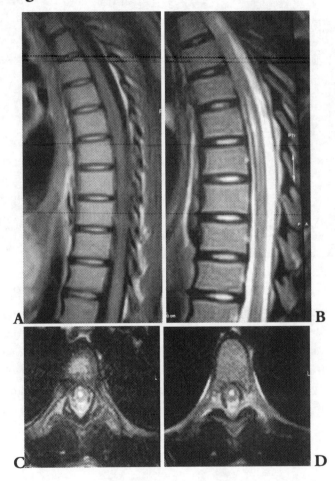

MR Scan, sagittal T1 (A), and sagittal (B) and axial (C, D)T2-weighted images showing a fusiform centro-medullary cystic cavity of low-T1 and high-T2 with smooth and regular margins at T5-T7 level. No other medullary or vertebral abnormality seen.

Diagnosis: Localized Hydromyelia

Case 186

Clinical Presentation

A 45 year-old female patient with dorso-lumbar scoliosis.

Radiological Findings

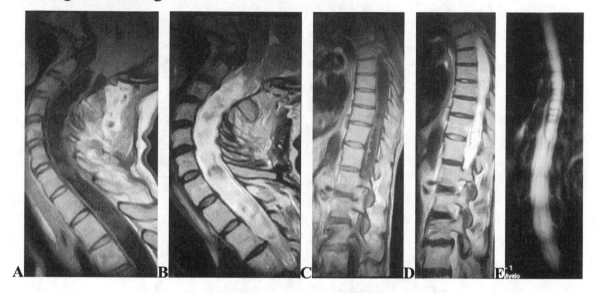

MR Scan of cervico-dorsal spine sagittal T1 (A, C) and T2 (B, D) with coronal myelo-MR-2D (E) images reveal a low position of the cerebellar tonsils in the foramen magnum indicating a tonsilar herniation. There is a Low-T1 and high-T2 well-defined, intra-medullary cystic lesion enlarging the spinal cord, extending from the bulbo-medullary junction up to conus medullary with no soft tissue component. The myelo-MR shows a thin septations within the cystic lesion giving a caterpillar appearance. Upward displacement with posterior angulation of the odontoid process indicating basilar impression with platybasia.

Diagnosis: Chiari I malformation with extensive Syringohydromyelia, Basilar Impression and Platybasia

Case 187

Clinical Presentation

A 39 year-old female patient presented with history of progressive tetraparesis.

Radiological Findings

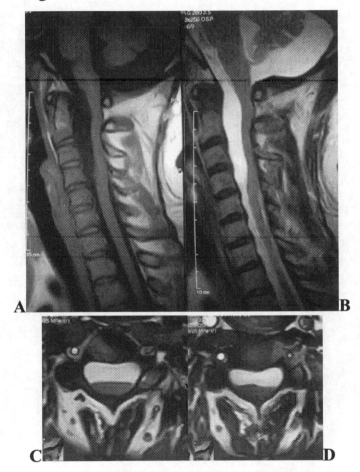

MR Scan, sagittal T1 (A), sagittal (B) and axial T2 (C, D) weighted images showing an intra-dural extra-medullary fusiform cystic mass with a signal intensity slightly higher than CSF on both sequences. This cystic lesion is of anterior location, extending from C1 to C4 level, compressing and displacing the bulbo-medullary junction and upper spinal cord posteriorly.

Diagnosis: Intra-spinal Arachnoid Cyst

Case 188

Clinical Presentation

An 18 year-old male patient with bilateral L5-S1 motor deficit and bladder dysfunction.

Radiological Findings

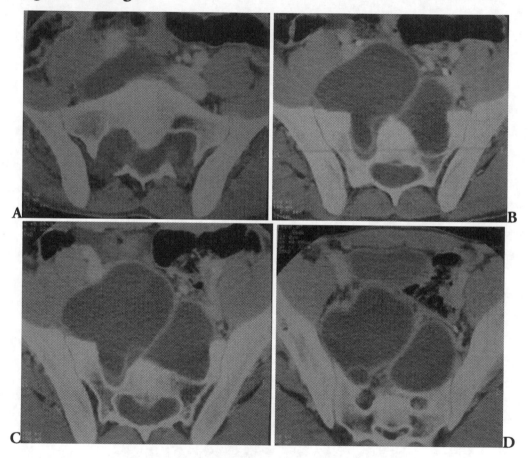

Post-contrast Sacral CT Scan showing an enlargement of the sacral canal and foramina by cystic lesions of CSF density with enhanced wall, presenting an anterior extension through a defect of the wall of the sacral foramina to the pelvic region compressing and displacing the bladder anteriorly.

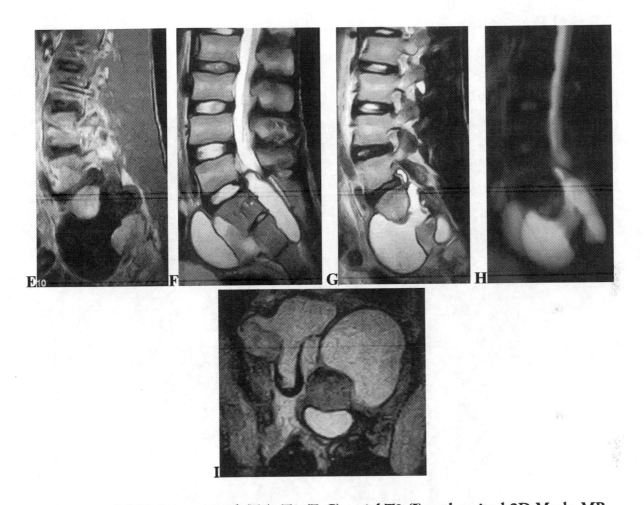

...continued, MR Scan sagittal (T1), T2 (F, G), axial T2 (I) and sagittal 2D Myelo-MR (H) showing an enlargement of the sacral canal by an intrasacral cystic lesion of CSF signal intensity with proper wall extending from L5-S1 to S2-S3 level, communicating with other similar cystic lesions of anterior presacral location through a defect of the sacral foramina.

Diagnosis : Intra- and Pre-sacral Meningocele

Case 189

Clinical Presentation

A 3 year-old male child with low lumbar mass.

Radiological Findings

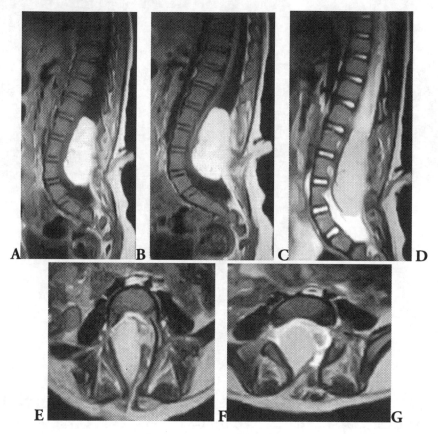

MR Scan, sagittal T1 (A, B) and T2 (C) and axial T2 (E, F) showing a large oval well-defined intra-canalar mass of fatty signal on both sequences, located posterior to the spinal cord which is tethered with a conus medullaris at L3-L4 level. There is a sinus tract seen as a linear hypointense structure crossing the subcutaneous tissue toward the spinal canal through the bifid spinous elements, to joint the low-lying tethered spinal cord.

Diagnosis: Dermal Sinus with Tethered Spinal Cord and Intra-spinal Lipoma

Case 190

Clinical Presentation

A 2 months old female child with posterior cervical mass.

Radiological Findings

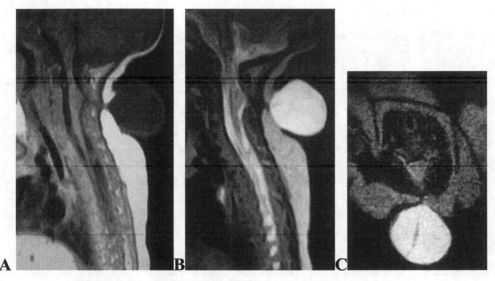

MR Scan, Sagittal T1 (A) and sagittal and axial T2 (B, C) weighted images showing a large oval median cystic mass of the posterior cervical region, not covered with skin, its signal is identical to that the CSF on both sequences T1 and T2, containing linear structure (neural tissue) isointense to the spinal cord. This cystic mass communicates with the spinal canal through an opened spinal dysraphism (spina bifida aperta) at C3 with triangular shape of the adjacent spinal cord segment pointing toward the spinal dysraphism. No abnormality of the posterior cerebral fossa.

Diagnosis: Cervical Myelomeningocele

Case 191

Clinical Presentation

A 30 year-old female patient with numerous cutaneous café au lait spots, presented with flask paraplegia.

Radiological Findings

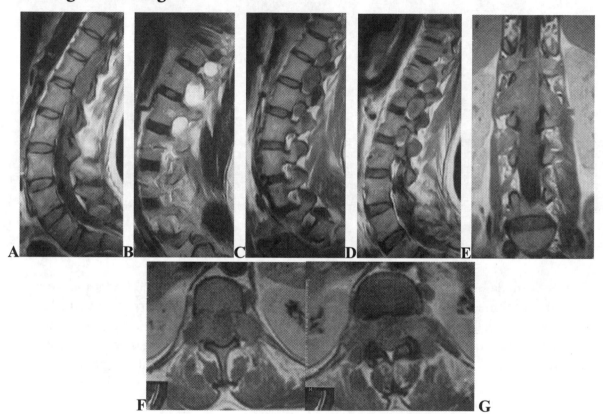

MR Scan, pre-contrast sagittal T1 (A), and T2 (B) and post-contrast sagittal (C, D), coronal (E) and axial (F, G) T1-weighted images showing multiple and bilateral intra-dural extra-medullary dumbbell lesions with intra-and extra-canalar location seen at several levels (from T11-T12 up to L1-L2), compressing the spinal cord, enlarging the adjacent foramina bilaterally with posterior vertebral scalloping. These lesions appear slightly hypointense to the spinal cord on T1 and hyperintense on T2 with moderate and heterogeneous enhancement after gadolinium administration. The coronal image shows the plexiform appearance of the lesions (neurofibromas).

Diagnosis: Von Recklinghausen's Disease (or Neurofibromatosis Type I)

Case 192

Clinical Presentation

A 27 year-old male patient, known case of trisomy 21, presented with tetraparesis..

Radiological Findings

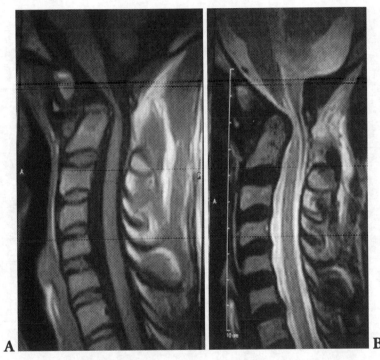

MR Scan sagittal T1 (A) and T2 (B) weighted images showing an increased distance between the anterior arch of C1 and odontoid process, indicating C1-C2 subluxation with hypoplasia of the odontoid process. Posterior angulation of C2 reducing the diameter of the foramen magnum and compressing severely the bulbo-medullary junction, which is atrophied with linear high-T2 intra-medullary areas indicating chronic myelopathy.

Diagnosis: Cervico-occipital Anomalies In Down's Syndrome

Case 193

Clinical Presentation

A 5 months old male child with posterior midline neck swelling.

Radiological Findings

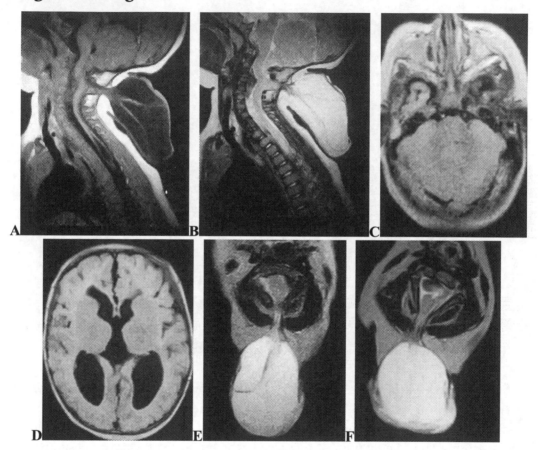

MR Scan, sagittal T1 (A), sagittal (B) and axial (E, F) T2 at the cervico-occipital region and axial FLAIR (C, D) of brain MR Scan, demonstrate a large posterior midline cervical mass with no skin cover, communicating with the spinal canal through an opened spinal dysraphism (spina bifida aperta); its signal is identical to that of CSF on both sequences T1 and T2, containing linear structures (neural tissue) isointense to the spinal cord with triangular shape of the adjacent spinal cord segment pointing toward the spinal dysraphism. Note herniation of the cerebellar tonsils through the foramen magnum with hydrosyringomyelia of the upper dorsal spinal cord. The 4th ventricle is laminated with dilated supra-tentorial ventricular system.

Diagnosis: Chiari III Malformation

Case 194

Clinical Presentation

A 12 year-old female patient presenting a bilateral peripheral neuropathy.

Radiological Findings

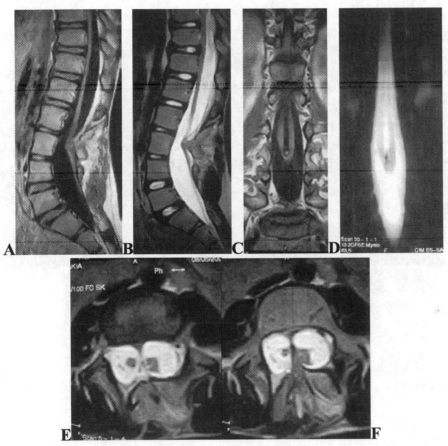

MR Scan, sagittal (A), and coronal (C) T1, sagittal (B) and axial (E, F)T2-weighted images and coronal Myelo-MR-2D (D): The lower spinal cord is clefted sagittally into two asymmetrical hemicords, separated by an osseous spur and each one is surrounded by the dural sac. Thin elongated lower spinal cord extending all the way down up to L5-S1 level with anterior ectasia of the dural sac. Spina bifia occulta at several levels.

Diagnosis: Diastematomyelia with Tethered Spinal Cord

Case 195

Clinical Presentation

An 18 months old male child presenting an urethral duplication and club feet. On the x-rays the thoracic vertebra are abnormal with enlarged canal.

Radiological Findings

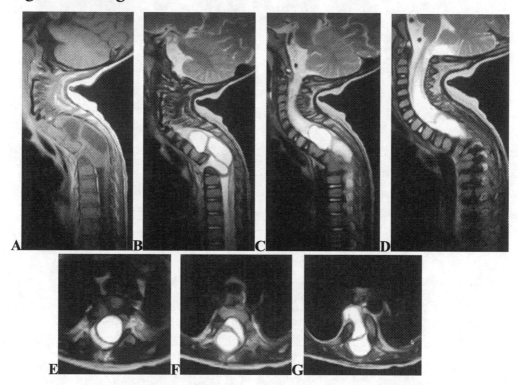

MR Scan, sagittal T1 (A), T2 (B, C, D) and axial T2 (E, F, G)-weighted images demonstrate an enlarged cervical spinal canal with an intra-medullary syringohydromyelic cavity enlarging the spinal cord from C2 up to T2 level, associated with a multiloculated intradural pre-medullary cystic mass of CSF signal intensity extending from T2 to T6 level, compressing and displacing the spinal cord dorsally. This cystic mass shows right pre-vertebral extension in the posterior mediastium through a corporeal defect of T6 "butterfly vertebra".

Diagnosis: Split Notochord Syndrome with Syringohydromyelia and Neuroenteric Cyst

Case 196

Clinical Presentation

An 8 months old female born with posterior lumbosacral mass.

Radiological Findings

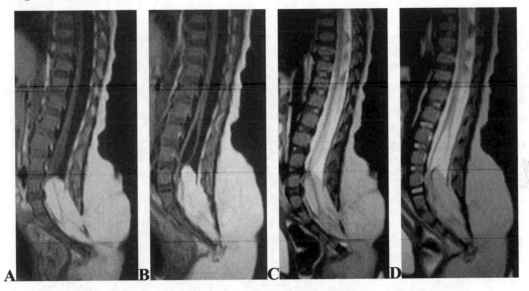

MR Scan, sagittal T1 (A, B) and T2 (C, D)-weighted images demonstrate a large posterior lumbosacral mass of high signal on T1 and reduced signal on T2 exactly as does the subcutaneous fat with intact skin cover; this mass extends into the canal through the spina bifida and appears attached to the dorsal surface of neural tissue. The spinal cord itself is tethered at L4-L5 level and showed a fusiform terminal cystic cavity of low-T1 and high T2 corresponding to a terminal ventricle.

Diagnosis: Lipomyelocele with Tethered Spinal Cord and Terminal Ventricle

Case 197

Clinical Presentation

A 6 months old female born with posterior lumbosacral mass.

Radiological Findings

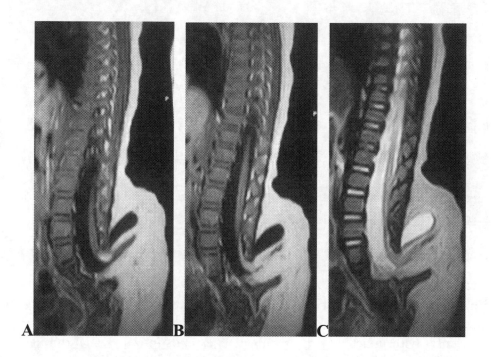

MR Scan, sagittal T1 (A, B) and T2 (C)-weighted images show a large posterior lumbosacral mass of fatty signal intensity exactly as the subcutaneous fat on both sequences, and extends into the spinal canal through the spina bifida and appears attached to the dorsal surface of spinal cord. This lumbosacral mass contains a cystic component of CSF signal intensity, communicating with the spinal subarachnoid spaces. The spinal cord itself is tethered and angulated posteriorly under the last intact lamina at the upper margin of the spina bifida

Diagnosis: Lipomyelomeningocele

Case 198

Clinical Presentation

A 6 months old male with posterior midline dorsal swelling since birth.

Radiological Findings

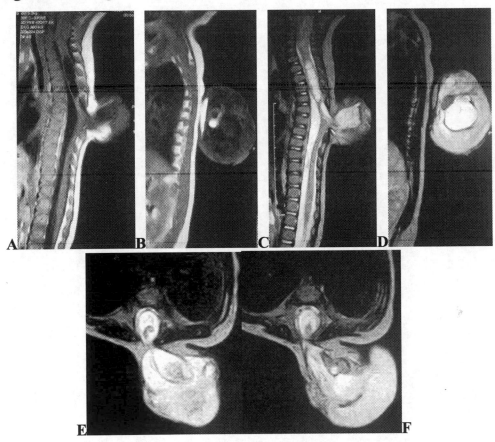

MR Scan, sagittal T1 (A, B), T2 (C, D) and axial T2 (E, F)-weighted images demonstrate a large posterior midline dorsal mass with no skin cover, communicating with the spinal canal through an opened spinal dysraphism (spina bifida aperta); its signal is identical to that of CSF on both sequences T1 and T2, containing linear structures (neural tissue) isointense to the spinal cord and a small fatty tissue area (intra-dural lipoma). Triangular shape of the adjacent spinal cord segment pointing toward the spinal dysraphism with syringohydromyelia and tonsilar herniation through the foramen magnum.

Diagnosis: Chiari II Malformation with Syringohydromyelia

Miscellaneous

Case 199

Clinical Presentation

A 26 year-old male patient, known case of heart disease under thrombolytic therapy, admitted for an acute paraplegia.

Radiological Findings

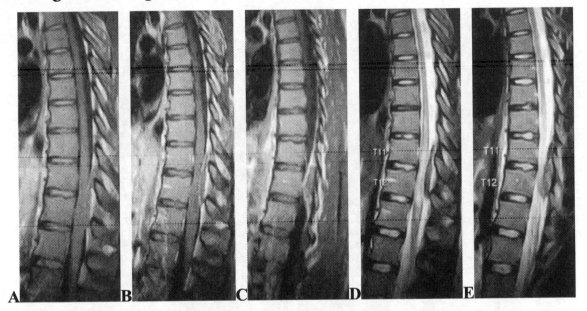

MR Scan, pre-(A) and post-contrast (B, C) sagittal T1 and sagittal T2 (D, E)-weighted images show a fusiform posterior epidural mass at T11-T12 level, isointense to the spinal cord on T1 and hypointense on T2 with no enhancement after gadolinium administration, compressing and displacing the lower spinal cord anteriorly which shows intra-medullary high-T2 areas indicating edema.

Diagnosis: Epidural Hematoma, Compressing the Spinal Cord

Case 200

Clinical Presentation

A 23 year-old male patient, operated twice for disc herniation at L4-L5 and L5-S1, actually complaining of localised low back pain.

Radiological Findings

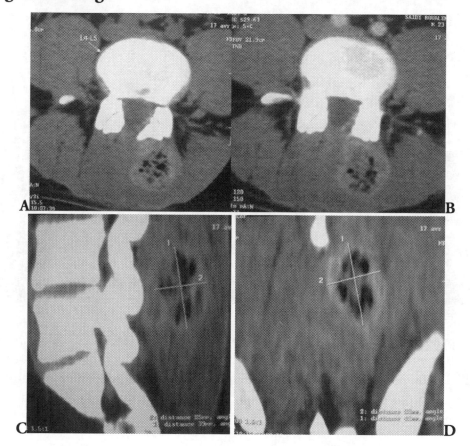

CT Scan of lumbar spine, pre(A)-and post-contrast (B) at L4-L5 level with sagittal (C) and coronal (D) reconstruction, reveals a mass lesion in the left posterior paravertebral region, containing air-bubbles with peripheral enhancement (thick fibrous capsule) at the level of the laminectomy.

Diagnosis: Textiloma (or Gossypiboma)

INDEX

A

abscess
  cerebellar, 45
  cerebral, 46-47
acoustic schwannoma, 120-21
acute
  disseminated encephalomyelitis, 50
  epidural hematoma, 33, 245
  subdural hematoma, 18
  transverse myelitis, 196-97
agenesis corpus callosum, 137-39
alobar holoprosencephaly, 142
aneurysm
  basilar artery, 30
  internal carotid artery (ICA), 28
  vein of Galen, 31
angioma
  cavernous, 22, 23, 24
  cerebral venous, 20-21
anoxo-ischemic encephalopathy, 16
aqueductal stenosis, 151
arachnoid cyst
  of cerebellopontine angle, 129
  of choroid fissure, 65
  intraspinal, 229
  intraventricular, 132
  with hydrocephalus, 130
  of quadrigeminal cistern, 133
  of the temporal fossa, 131
arachnoiditis, 195
arterio-venous malformation, 27, 223
astrocytoma
  brainstem, 62
  cerebellar, 72-74
  in spinal cord, 177-78
  in tuberous sclerosis, 161

atrophy
  cerebellar, 57
  cerebral, 58

B

Basilar impression, 224, 228
brachial plexus avulsion, 209
brainstem
  astrocytoma, 62
  glioma, 62, 77, 79
  stroke, 4-5
brucellar spondylodiscitis, 191

C

callosal agenesis, 137-39, 147
carcinoma nasopharyngeal, 126
Caudal Regression Syndrome, 217
Cavernous Angioma, 22, 23, 24
cavity, postoperative, 81
cerebellar
  abscess, 45
  astrocytoma, 75
  atrophy, 57
  hemangioblastoma, 71
cerebral
  astrocytoma, 75
  abscess, 46-47
  atrophy, 58
  contusion, 34
  hydatid cyst, 49
  lymphoma, 91
  metastases, 66-67
  vein thrombosis, 19
  venous angioma, 20-21
Chiari I malformation, 62, 154, 219, 224, 228

Chiari II malformation, 156, 241
Chiari III malformation, 157, 236
Choroid Plexus Papilloma, 68-69
colloid cyst of third ventricle, 76
cord injury, 209-12
craniopharyngioma, 119
cyst
   arachnoid, 65, 129-33
   dermoid, 124-25
   epidermoid, 111-12, 134-35
   neuroenteric, 238
   Rathke's cleft, 136
   third ventricle colloid, 76
Cystic Glioblastoma, 85

D

dermal sinus, 232
dermoid cyst
   quadrigeminal cistern, 124
   sellar and suprasellar, 125
diastematomyelia, 237
disc herniation
   cervical, 201-2
   dorsal, 203
   lumbar, 204-205
dislocation of the spine, 213
Down's syndrome, 235
Dural Arteriovenous Malformation (DAVM), 32

E

empyema, 48
encephalitis, 43-44
encephalomalacia, 15
encephalopathy anoxo-ischemic, 16
ependymoma of the fourth ventricle, 63, 65
epidermoid cyst
   of cerebello-pontine angle (CPA), 134
   intradiploic, 111-12
   of temporal fossa, 135
Extradural Empyema, 48

F

fibrous dysplasia, 113
fistula
   osteo-dural, 39
   spinal dural arteriovenous (SDAVF), 223

fracture of the spine, 213

G

Galen's vein aneurysm, 31
ganglioglioma, 87
germinoma, 70
glioblastoma, 82-85
glioma in the brainstem, 62, 77, 79
gliomatosis cerebri, 86
gossypiboma, 246

H

hemangioblastoma cerebellar, 71
hemangioma vertebral, 185
hematoma
   acute subdural, 18
   chronic subdural, 36-37
   epidural, 245
   extradural, 33
   retroclival, 25
   subacute subdural, 35
hemorrhagic
   infarct, 19
   stroke, 17-18
heterotopia
   subcortical, 147
   subependymal, 65, 139, 148
histiocytosis X, 168, 184
holoprosencephaly alobar, 142
hydatid cyst
   in the brain, 49
   in the spine, 193
hydrocephalus, 69, 73, 76, 130, 152, 154, 161, 219
hydromyelia, 227
hydrosyringomyelia, 219, 224, 241
hygroma
   subarachnoid, 208
   subdural, 38

I

infarction
   anterior cerebral artery (ACA) territory, 13
   brainstem, 4-5
   middle cerebral artery (MCA) territory, 8-9, 11-12, 14

posterior ceberal artery (PCA) territory, 6
vertebrobasilar territory, 7
injury cord, 209, 213
Ischemic Myelopathy, 198

J

Joubert's syndrome, 150

L

leukemia, 182
lipoma
    Interpeduncular, 140
    interhemispheric, 138
    intraspinal, 225-26, 232
    quadrigeminal cistern, 141
lipomyelocele, 239
lipomyelomeningocele, 240
lissencephaly, 144
lymphoma cerebral, 91

M

macroadenoma, 116, 118
macroprolactinoma, 117
malformative scoliosis, 221-22
meningioma
    cavernous sinus, 99
    cerebello-pontine angle (CPA), 94
    of cerebral convexity, 106
    en plaque, 108-9
    of the falx cerebri, 107
    at the foramen magum, 93
    frontal, 100-101
    of the jugum, 102
    olfactory groove, 95, 97
    of the optic gutter, 102
    of the pineal region, 104
    retroclival, 110
    sphenoid wing, 105
    of the thoracic spine, 173
meningocele
    intra-and presacral 230
    occipital, 153
Mesial Temporal Sclerosis (MTS), 149
metastases
    brain, 66-67

subarachnoid, 181
vertebral, 179-80
microadenoma, 114-15
multiple sclerosis, 51, 53
myelitis
    acute transverse, 196-97
    tuberculous (TB), 195
myelomeningocele,
    cervical 233
    lumbar, 156, 220
myelopathy
    compressive, 218
    ischemic, 198

N

Nasopharyngeal Carcinoma, 126
neuroenteric cyst, 238
neurofibromatosis
    type 1, *163, 234*
    type 2, *164, 166*

O

oligodendroglioma
    grade A, 89
    grade B, 90
osteodural fistula, 39

P

pachygyria, 143
papilloma choroid plexus, 68-69
paraganglioma, 122-23
peripheral primitive neuroectodermal tumor
    (PNET), 183
perisylvian polymicrogyria, 145
pilocytic astrocytoma, 75
polymicrogyria, 145
Postoperative Cavity, 81
pyogenic spondylodiscitis, 192

R

radionecrosis, 92
Rathke's cleft cyst, 136

S

schizencephaly, 146
schwannoma
   acoustic, 120-21
   cervical, 174
   thoracic, 175-76
scoliosis, 221
spinal
   cord injury, 210
   dislocation, 213
   hydatidosis, 193
Spinal Dural Arteriovenous Fistula (SDAVF), 223
split notochord syndrome, 238
spondylodiscitis
   Brucellar, 191
   pyogenic, 192
   tuberculous (TB), 189-90
spondylolisthesis, 206-7
stenosis aqueductal, 151
Sturge-Weber syndrome, 159
subarachnoid
   hygroma, 208
   metastasis, 181
subcortical heterotopia, 147
subdural hematoma
   chronic, 36-37
   subacute, 35
subdural hygroma, 38
subependymal heterotopia, 64-65, 139, 148
syringohydromyelia, 228, 238, 241
syrinx, 218

T

terminal ventricle, 239
tethered cord, 220, 225-26, 232, 237, 239
Textiloma, 246
thrombosis
   basilar artery aneurysm, 30
   cerebral venous sinus (CVST), 19
tuberous sclerosis, 160-161

V

vein of Galen aneurysm, 31
Venous Angioma, 20-21
vertebral
   hemangioma, 185
   malformation, 221, 224
   metastases, 179-80
Von Recklinghausen's disease, 163, 234

W

Wallenberg syndrome, 3